KIDNEYS, CRAZINESS & COURAGE

Leading to Hope And Help for Kidney Failure

To Jim, a great concierge

from Peter

To Jim, a great
concierge
from Peter

KIDNEYS, CRAZINESS & COURAGE

Leading to Hope And Help for Kidney Failure

Dr. Peter Cohen, PhD, and
Chrissy Meade, BA

Library of Congress Control Number: 2011908671
ISBN: Hardcover   978-1-4628-7879-6
               Softcover   978-1-4628-7878-9
               Ebook   978-1-4628-7880-2

This book was printed in the United States of America.

To order additional copies of this book, contact:
Xlibris Corporation
1-888-795-4274
www.Xlibris.com
Orders@Xlibris.com
97391

Contents

Foreword 9

Kidneys, Craziness, Courage, and Drink for His Dear Ones 11

1. Courage: One Way to Realize and Nurture It 13
2. My Dear Ones: My Work on Skid Row 17
3. The Twelve Steps of Alcoholics Anonymous 33
4. Rational-Emotive Therapy of Alcoholism 34
5. Chrissy's Song 35
6. My Experience With Barbara 40
7. Happy Endings 53

PART 2
HOPE AND HELP FOR KIDNEY FAILURE

1. Hope and Help for Kidney Failure–Abstract 65
2. Introduction 67
3. Review of the Literature 71
4. Procedures 89
5. Results and Summary 91
6. Appendix: Hope and Help for Kidney Failure 95
7. Kidney Failure and Its Treatment 97
8. Causes of Chronic Renal Failure 104
9. Other Treatments for Kidney Failure and Coping
   with Kidney Failure 114
10. Future of Kidney-Failure Research 132

Bibliography 145

THIS BOOK IS DEDICATED TO DIANE DIAMOND

Foreword

Peter Cohen's leading aim was to learn how to live in life, how to last, and (having lasted) how to use a carefully cultivated stoical fortitude to improve the well-being of others. The following words will help you to comprehend, a little, the concept of Peter Cohen. There is, first, the immensely ambitious young man, unfailingly competitive, driven by an urge to excel in anything he undertook to be admired and looked up to, to assert his superiority by repeated example, to display for the benefit of others his strength and his endurance. The very same man who displays his hatred of diabetes, kidney failure, cancer, heart disease, and leukemia; his rulership over fear and pain; and his proud defiance of death.

There is, next, the man of many contradictions: the shy and diffident man and the incredible braggart; the tremendously warm, loving, and affectionate man and the man given to tremendous hatred; the non-hero longing for hero status and sometimes achieving it; the man of action harnessed to the same chariot as the man of words; and the author who impugned all cheap and easy writing yet boiled as many pots as the next man before he was through. There is the perpetual student, the omnivorous reader, and the brilliant health scientist. There is the romantic liar for whom the line between fact and fiction was thinner than a hair and who sometimes embellished some of his achievements.

There is the man driven by pride—sometimes defined as a deadly sin but which he embraced as his personal and well-beloved demon. He was proud of his manhood, his literary and athletic skills, his staying and recuperative powers, his title, his earnings, his medical and psychological knowledge, and a few other skills. There is the temperamental paranoia schizophrenic, the inveterate hypochondriac and valetudinarian who seriously contemplated suicide at times in his life, yet possessed of enormous powers of resilience and recuperation that could bring him from the brink to the peak within days or sometimes even hours. He was a persistent worrier who wryly cautioned others against this most pernicious habit. He was plagued all his adult life by tormenting thoughts and feelings, partly the product of a highly developed imagination.

There was the muscular physique, athletic and fit, often ingratiating and impressive to some people. He was five foot six and weighed about 155 pounds. He had a tendency to put on weight and was once up to 191 pounds. His eyes were hazel and his complexion ruddy, his head bald with salt-and-pepper hair on the sides and back.

He is said, by those who know, to have been a perfectly satisfactory lover without being a Don Juan. He formed many friendships with women, both older and younger, and considered himself to be defined by his romantic and sexual attraction to women. The main love of his life was Diane who was with him for eighteen years. He admired courage and stoical endurance in women as in men and disliked hard back talk.

In his treatment of those he liked or loved, there was often something of the chivalric; although sometimes, when angered, he could be excessively cruel and abusive.

He is one of the most original health scientists Canada has produced, a powerful inventor of new techniques and ideas. He is interesting both as a man of action and a professional.

Kidneys, Craziness, Courage, and Drink for His Dear Ones

This is the story of Diane and I and our fight against kidney failure. I was the crazy one; Diane was the kidney patient.

My life started in a warm, loving way. The one problem was that our housemates' father used to get drunk and dash me into the ground. He later went to jail.

All through my younger years, I had been a good student and a good athlete. I was small, wiry, and fast. I also wet the floor several times because I was too shy to ask to be excused. I continued to play football and compete in boxing until I got too badly injured.

Moving on to more important matters—to my friend Diane, her modest life, and her courageous death. Diane was a very special woman who brought great joy to her parents and sisters and later to me. She was like the ugly duckling who turned into the beautiful swan. Diane was born with Bardet-Biedl syndrome, a rare genetic disorder associated with intellectual problems, deformed hands and feet, motivational problems, obesity, and diabetes. Diabetes was the main cause of her early death at the tender age of fifty. She went into acute respiratory distress syndrome after inhaling some vomit.

In Diane's younger years, she had the benefit of a loving family—first her parents, then her sisters. Her father came up through the concentration camps and came to Canada poor. Through courage and perseverance, he built up tremendous wealth. Her mother was also poor when she was young. I remember Diane's parents to be warm and generous.

Diane was in many ways a bright woman who could rise to the occasion. She had excellent conversational skills. She carried the conversation when my cousins came over for dinner. Diane was like the song "Honey." She was always young at heart and kinda dumb and kinda smart, and I loved her so.

Diane showed great personal courage in overcoming her fear of needles and problems associated with dialysis in order to keep herself alive. She showed "grace under pressure" in many situations. This is in keeping with my existentialist psychology that it takes courage just to live.

Another person who showed great courage was Mr. Chan. He had emigrated to Canada from Hong Kong and worked very hard at clerical work in spite of a stroke that made him type more slowly. He was very gracious in handling his dialysis and various problems that came up.

Bill Einarson showed great courage in facing open-heart surgery without showing any signs of fear. He blew me away.

Isaak Moldaver was one of my favorites. He put up with dialysis, nausea, and the pain of surgery with no complaint. He was so generous that he would give away some of his food and the shirt off his back. Before he got sick, he worked out at the "Y" for three hours, four times per week. The greatest, I will save for later.

Courage: One Way to Realize and Nurture It

Some of what I will now describe is dangerous, stupid, and useless. Please do not attempt to try it. I am extremely fortunate to be alive. I now believe that I am a good and decent man and would never do the following dangerous stunts again. However, courage itself is a marvelous quality.

The first step towards developing courage is to list your past achievements and build confidence in yourself. Next, list things that you would like to accomplish. Third, list steps needed to reach that goal. The next step is to put your ideas into action, one by one. It is better to try to develop moral courage over putting your life on the line unnecessarily. I stopped dangerous stunts at age twenty. By the way, if your goal is combat, relaxation training is very helpful.

Some Definitions of Courage

One of my heroes, Ernest Hemingway, defined courage as "grace under pressure." This is my favorite definition provided that you are doing something useful.

John McCain, US senator, said, "Do not take fear as a sign of cowardice. By accepting the fear and using our actions for good, we will show love. Love is useful to everyone." Scott Peck, MD, defined love as "a will to extend yourself to improve someone's mind or spirit." I think that courage and love are closely related. General Sherman defined courage as "a willingness to stay in a position that we feel fear."

Another author says that courage is conscience turned outward onto the environment.

Developing Courage

1.   Improve strength and endurance. (Il faut d'abord durer, meaning "it is necessary at first to last.")

2.   Practice courage, especially when your life is not in danger.

3.   Develop skills and interests.

4.   Love all people, and also a special person.

5.   Visualize yourself being courageous.

6.   Want to have courage.

7.   Pray for courage.

8.   Do mental and physical exercises like self-hypnosis.

9.   Care about people around you.

10. Think about being brave and tough and act it.

11. Write down your accomplishments and make goals.

12. Do muscle relaxation, sensory awareness, and stress inoculation training. Remember that discretion is the better part of valour.

Examples

1.   I led canoe trips for three years, shot rapids, and carried canoes over anything.

2.   I boxed from age seventeen to age twenty.

3.   I played football for three years.

4.   I did chin-ups and hangs from various high bridges twenty or thirty times.

5.   I went against advice and got straight A's from a science course at Wilfrid Laurier.

6.   I took a job working with alcoholics, against advice. I stood up to their assault, bottle throwing, and other "fun."

7.   I went to nursing school. This is good for anyone.

8.   Asking girls for dates sometimes takes courage.

9.   I stood up to a man who assaulted people.

10.   I overcame agoraphobia.

11.   I helped a prostitute get away from a gun-toting madman.

12.   I got my PhD.

12.   I held my forearm against a steaming hot kettle for fifteen minutes, resulting in a severe watery blister that took several months to heal. I just smiled through it all.

13.   I wrote a scathing report on a wife-and-child abuser and stood by it.

14.   I ran 32.8 miles in six hours and swam 5 miles in three hours.

15.   I stuck with my girlfriend through thick and thin.

16.   I served in the Canadian militia.

17.   I worked on a dangerous Israeli kibbutz.

18.   I took part in a research study at the Clarke Institute.

19.   I wrote a book called *From Mad to Glad*.

20.   I wrote several magazine articles.

21. I saved several lives over my professional career.

22. I helped rehabilitate several people.

23. I made people more comfortable.

24. I helped some people die more comfortably.

The Greatest of All: My Dad

I look on myself as someone who was pushed out of harm's way by a brave heart, namely my dad. He was mentally strong and could probably give emotional support to half the world. Above all, Dad was a family man. He worked harder than anyone I knew and frequently put in eighteen hours, six days a week. He overcame his anxiety about supporting the family and was always present like a rock for advice or support. Dad worked full-time until his final illness.

The story of my father swimming out to rescue someone is not well-known, but he could have been killed himself. Dad completed his courage by showing stoical endurance when having painful dental procedures and not being stopped by pain. Everyone loved him, but especially his family.

My Dear Ones:
My Work on Skid Row

"You — Jew, you're going to get your head punched in. You'll be taken care of," said the man as he got up to attack me.

In another incident, I had just taken a bottle of liquor from someone, and as I turned to empty it, a bottle of Canadian sherry came flying past my ear. I cleaned up the glass and got out as quickly as possible. The man later apologized and explained that he could not control himself when he was drinking. He explained that one of his biggest problems was that he suffered remorse caused by his drunken behaviour. We later became close friends, and he always made an effort to tone down his excesses even when he was drunk, although his drinking never stopped. The man from the previous incident also became friendly once physiotherapy gave him hope for a better life. He had previously been friendly, and I will always think of him as his good self.

"Your work with me has given me a new lease on life," said another man.

"Thanks a lot for your help, I feel a lot better now," said a man that I had just cleaned up.

These are anecdotes that show that working with alcoholics and skid row people can be very demanding and also very rewarding. The good far outweighed the bad, and the residents of the mission became very dear to me. In the following pages, I will tell of my work with skid row people, set straight some myths and truisms, show some of the humorous and possibly adventurous aspects of working in the home, and hopefully enrich your life as these men have enriched mine. These men were graduates of "the college of hard knocks" and taught me a great deal about handling life. They were tough, but kind. They often used foul language, but it usually was not malicious—meaning not directed towards people.

The Origin of the Term "Skid Row"

The term "skid row" came from early logging days, about late 1800s or early 1900s. Loggers would come into town and need a place to stay. Wealthy individuals (in conjunction with religious organizations) would start missions to give lost, uncared-for people—sometimes called "derelicts"—a place to stay. Many of the people staying in missions were loggers and had travelled into town on logs as if they had skid along the logs. They called the travelling along these logs "skid road" because the loggers skid along the logs. This later evolved into "skid row," just like a prison for people waiting to die is called "death row." Skid row did not originally mean people who had skid to rock bottom, as some people believed.

It is also important to point out that working with alcoholics and skid row people is not bad, as some people believe. Before I took the job at the mission, a number of people warned me not to take the job because working with skid row alcoholics was just too difficult. I was certainly pleasantly surprised. This job was my first full-time job after graduating university, and at first, I took it because I was desperate. But I soon came to enjoy it immensely. We had a great bunch of residents, outstanding supervisors to work under, and a chance to make a difference in the lives of the residents. It gave meaning to my life. This was another reason why the residents were very dear to me. In addition, the money that I earned helped me to further my education as it became painfully evident that I needed upgrading for that job.

The Mission and Its Purpose

The mission was founded by a religious group in conjunction with a wealthy family and several donations in order to provide food and shelter to men who otherwise would not be cared for. One side of the mission was for transients, mostly younger, but some were older men who needed a place to provide food and shelter. The side of the mission that I worked on was a home for older men. These men were referred by the hostel for transients, various hospitals and agencies, and any place aware of the mission's services. Ironically, one man was referred to the mission from a hospital after suffering scurvy. He could have gone to another place, but our mission was chosen because it did not allow drinking. It turned out that the majority of the men in the home were heavy drinkers, and the garbage cans were filled to the brim with empty liquor bottles. About two-thirds of the residents were active drinkers, and several others had had experience with alcohol and either did not drink, or drank seldom. Some residents had never drunk at all. There were very few who did not smoke, and it seemed a miracle that many of these men lived into their eighties and sometimes nineties. I wondered if this was due to the toughness of the residents or the fact that they did not worry much or, even more likely, natural selection—meaning that the strong survive.

Our purpose was not to treat the alcoholism but to provide a good place for the men to stay, to provide good health care and hygiene, and provide food and shelter. These factors tended to minimize the harmful effects of drinking. The men who did not stop drinking did not want to stop.

The administrator was a minister, and to this day, I have never worked for a finer man. He was always very kind and generous, eager to listen, and helpful with both personal problems and problems related to work. One of the residents remarked that when they made Mr. Martin they threw away the plans. That is probably why I have never had a boss that good again. He always made a point of telling people when they did a good job and was very diplomatic when correcting someone's mistake. This was the right way to handle people, and he was a master at handling people. A study done showed that people were able to find a specific object much more quickly when cheered as they got closer to the object than when they were booed when they got farther away from the object. In other words, positive reinforcement is a better motivator than negative reinforcement. Mr. Martin always had a great sense of humor and excellent courage in dealing with dangerous situations, such as when a violent non-resident would enter the home. He was also humble enough to do any task such as washing the floor, hanging drapes, or waiting on the men with food.

The head nurse, who supervised me more directly because of her medical knowledge, was every bit as good as Mr. Martin in her own way. She had a wealth of knowledge that came from forty years in the nursing profession. Four and a half of those years were as a head nurse in intensive care. She was not only good at dealing with people, both patients and staff, but she could spot problems early in their development and prevent them from becoming more serious. For example, one man had deep vein thrombosis—a clot in the large veins in the leg. Dorothy, the head nurse, spotted that something was seriously wrong and sent him to the hospital. He was given anticoagulants that probably saved his life. Blood clots in deep veins can be thrown into circulation and damage the brain, heart, and lungs and kill the person. Dorothy showed great courage in disarming a man with a switchblade when he went to stab another resident in order to gain money for drinking. The man with the switchblade had earlier told me that he would not hesitate to cut someone's throat because he was eighty-four and could not be put in jail for long. The man was later thrown out and sent to a nursing home, where he died.

The home had one orderly on duty in the daytime, one in the evening, and one at night. The head nurse worked Monday to Friday, from eight to four. One orderly was a doctor from Hong Kong who was waiting to pass his Canadian licensing exams. The other orderly was someone with a registered nursing assistant diploma from Nova Scotia. There was another orderly who had worked in hospitals for twenty years and had picked up a great deal of knowledge. The man who usually did nights was an engineering school dropout. In spite of his lack of medical knowledge, he had common sense and good judgment and could handle the emergencies that arose. The staff was competent and caring, except for me.

My own training, at the time, was a premedical degree with an emphasis on psychology, science, and health science. I was very enthusiastic and constantly tried to upgrade myself. I certainly needed it. I first took the health care aide program, but that was not enough. I audited the paramedic course at a local community college, but it was not until I studied nursing at University of Toronto that I felt that I knew enough to look after the residents. The men had many serious medical problems that could cause them a lot of danger very quickly. As I mentioned, I got a lot of help from the Chinese doctor and the head nurse. I forgot to mention that we had an orderly for a few weeks who was drunk more often than the residents. He used to confiscate the residents' liquor bottles and drink them himself. I was glad when he was fired.

Most of the men were getting old-age pensions or disability pensions, and they received a portion of this every month as "comfort money." The other portion of the residents' pensions went to running the home. Every payday (for the residents) at the first of the month, many residents would invest their money in alcohol and stay drunk until they ran out of money, usually a week or two after payday. They would be broke and sober for two to three weeks every month. Any time that they could get their hands on money, they would go right back to drinking. One of the men suffered seizures as a result of alcohol withdrawal, but most of the men functioned well without alcohol. There were no cases of delirium tremens, which is hallucinations caused by alcohol withdrawal, although some of the men reported previously experiencing that problem. There were many men who suffered brain damage from drinking and became very confused about where they were, who they were, what they were doing, and what was happening in the present. This disorder is an alcoholic psychosis called Korsakoff's syndrome because it was described by a Russian named Korsakoff. These unfortunate men did not always have an accurate perception of reality, which is a kind of definition of psychosis, and many of the victims knew what was wrong.

For example, one man said, "I used to be smart, but my mind is shot from drinking too much." It usually takes years of heavy drinking for Korsakoff's syndrome to develop.

I do not fully understand why we had a lot of heavy drinkers in our home, but maybe it was because the men who were drawn to the home had problems that they tried to solve with alcohol. In doing a study of alcoholism, I found that different people drink for different reasons, but they all had some problem that they were trying to solve. We could have ten drinkers in one room and they all might have different reasons for drinking. Drinking should not be looked down on. These men were the backbone of our country. Many of them were veterans. They worked hard, and they played hard. I had a great deal of respect for the men in the home. Some people are unfortunate to become alcoholics because they took a drink, liked it, and wanted to continue on. There is a theory put forth by an addiction counselor that I talked to that alcoholics have a different brain chemistry, which makes them enjoy drinking. I was fortunate that I never liked to drink, but I always said to myself and others, "There but for the grace of God go I."

Most of the men, with some exceptions, were likeable drunks.

Incidents and Anecdotes

"You don't have to be crazy to work here, but it helps."

This was a sign that I saw on the nursing station of a hospital ward. That would apply to our mission as well. As mentioned earlier, I had a great deal of respect for the men in the home. Nevertheless, they say the darnedest things that can be construed as funny if someone has a good sense of humor. The administrator had a good sense of humor and encouraged us to follow him.

One time, there was a fight between two residents. Mr. Martin described it, saying that Mr. Swanson, who was a confused man, tried to pick up someone's glasses because he thought they belonged to him. Mr. Iluha intervened and said that those were Jimmy's glasses. Everything else normal (Gerry had been drinking). Gerry was a leading alcoholic with Korsakoff's syndrome that I described earlier. He could be very funny at times. Every time he drank, he would say, "Mr. Martin was a boxer, and he said to me, 'Gerry, if I catch you drinking, I'm going to punch you right in the nose.'" Mr. Martin was a gentle man and would have been unlikely to punch anybody.

This man, Gerry Perk, was formerly a talented artist but was paid for his work in drinks because that was all that anyone could afford. In this way, he became an alcoholic. Gerry was always telling people that he worked hard all day long, painting. In reality, he had been sitting downstairs doing nothing, with a faraway look in his eyes. He would frequently come up to Mr. Martin and ask if he could pay for some food. Mr. Martin would always set him straight and say, "Everyone knows Gerry Perk. You've been here for years. Don't worry about food or rent, you're always paid up."

Gerry would say, "Do you know me?"

Mr. Martin would say, "Like a book."

Gerry would frequently come and ask what room he was in, and before he had a chance to say anything, we would say, "It's 207, Gerry."

He would walk away puzzled, wondering how we knew what he was going to ask. Gerry Perk was a likeable man.

Mr. Martin normally detested swearing. One time, when he was helping a drunk Gerry Perk to his bed, Mr. Perk said to Mr. Martin, "You're a fuck of a good head."

I think that Mr. Martin made an exception about swearing in those circumstances. Gerry Perk showed that he appreciated someone caring about him.

Gerry was sometimes afraid of his roommate, who would sometimes get violent when he got drunk. He'd go to Mr. Martin and say, "That fellow next to me, he's a big man. I don't want any trouble."

Mr. Martin would say, "He's just a little guy. You just have to blow on him and he'll fall apart."

In reality, the man was tiny and weak. Gerry would come back and say, "I don't care how small he is. I still don't want any trouble, and he seems to want to fight all the time." We would usually send him up to sick bay until his roommate sobered up.

One of my responsibilities was to look after the residents' personal hygiene such as baths, shaves, and dressing in clean clothes. I went to one man with a change of clothes and told him that I was going to give him a bath. He said, "I just had a bath."

I asked, "When was the last time you had a bath?"

He said, "It was only a month ago."

Eventually, he got a bath after Mr. Martin applied some pressure. Mr. Watson, the man who got the bath, said, "You had to keep bothering me."

Another man who did not want to have a bath cursed me with about every word in the book. After applying some pressure with help from Mr. Martin, we got him a bath and a change of clothes. He said, "Thanks a lot. I feel much better now."

James Watson would often get up in the middle of the night and state, "I've got to go look after my daughter and grandchildren."

The man next to him would keep up a running commentary, saying, "Can't even look after yourself, for Christ's sake."

One night, Mr. Watson woke up at 3 AM and stated that he wanted to go fishing. I don't know what made him say that.

Another time, I caught a man drinking a bottle of alcohol. I told him that we did not allow liquor in the home. He told me to go get the security guard to take away the bottle and that he would not touch a drop until I got back. I went downstairs to get the security guard, and when we came up the bottle was half empty, and he was pouring it down for all he was worth. The security guard confiscated what was left of the bottle. A few days later, when this man's best friend died, I said, "I'm terribly sorry, Mr. Sanchez."

He said, "That's okay. I didn't want to drink it, anyways."

He did not seem to realize that I was consoling him on the death of his friend.

Meet the Residents: My Dear Ones

One of the greatest joys in life is to help make someone's life a little better. One of the greatest disappointments in life is to fail in this regard. I experienced both on skid row. Here are some case histories that will help to give some idea what the men in the mission were really like.

The first case history that I will discuss is Mr. Frank Sanchez. I became very attached to him—partly because he was a kind, unselfish man and partly because he needed a lot of care.

One thing that illustrates how unselfish he was occurred after dinner one day. Mr. Sanchez had always had difficulty moving around—partly from taking haloperidol, an antipsychotic drug, and partly due to some injuries to his knees and hips. I came up, and Mr. Sanchez told me that he had used the wastebasket to defecate in because he did not want to make more work for us by messing the bed. This required considerable effort on his part, but as health care workers, we are not looking to have things made easier for us. We are mostly interested in patient welfare.

Even when Mr. Sanchez was dying of stomach cancer, he never complained. When I asked him how he was, he would always say, "Can't kick."

When he was annoyed, he would always say that he wouldn't know when asked how he was.

Frank Sanchez was a big, powerful man when he was in his prime. He emigrated from Spain in his early years and was a veteran of World War Two. After that, he became a lumberjack and a taxicab driver until he retired and came into our mission. He had some mobility deficits, and it was hard to get him to move. Frequently, he had to be cleaned. When he started to have fears of someone stabbing him with a knife, the doctor put him on large doses of an antipsychotic drug: haloperidol. He eventually became so immobile that he could not even roll over in bed and had to be positioned and have his clothing changed often. Even then, he was still uncomfortable a good part of the time. After he was taken off the haloperidol, he could walk with the assistance of a cane and did not have significant mobility problems until his cancer progressed to the terminal stages.

Mr. Sanchez was operated on for a benign prostate enlargement and was incontinent for a while after that. At one point, he stopped eating, and after several days of this, he finally asked to go to the hospital. When I phoned the hospital, I asked how Mr. Sanchez was, and the nurse replied that he was a very sick man and that his blood work was all abnormal. Eventually, we found out that he had cancer of the stomach, which had spread to several other organs. The doctor removed some of the cancer from his stomach and closed him up. The doctor also took him off haloperidol, which caused withdrawal symptoms so that Frank felt that he could not sleep for several days. After a while, he got used to being on no medication and could sleep, walk about, and had no sign of any particular emotional problems. Our head nurse decided that none of us should tell him that he was going to die and that he could enjoy six to eight months of good living.

Mr. Sanchez did very well for a few months, not drinking but still smoking. He enjoyed life and talked about the days he used to play baseball and do heavy construction work. After about five months, he started to go downhill and could not keep food down. I brought him some Kaiser rolls as he said that he would enjoy them. He continued to vomit and lose weight. He also asked for oxycodone to control his "aches and pains," which we were glad to supply. He continued to go downhill and asked to be taken to the hospital again. Our doctor told him that there was no point in further surgery as the cancer had spread throughout his body and he would not live more than two to three weeks.

Frank was very angry and said, "I'm going to have a long rest," meaning that he was going to die. I tried to see to his needs as best I could, changing his clothes and spending much time with him. At one point, he asked me to squeeze his fingers as they were cold. He probably had a mixture of fear and anger but always managed to smile in spite of the pain, which I am told is similar to a knife going through you. In the final stages, he had diarrhea and could not move because of the pain, so he needed to be cleaned up often. His skin was raw from stool and pressure on his bony skin. I cleaned him up one night and went to make rounds. When I came back fifteen minutes later, Mr. Sanchez was lying there, stiff, with his eyes rolled back in his head and having no pulse or respiration. I called an ambulance, and he was pronounced dead on arrival. He was sorrowfully missed by those who knew him.

Mr. Jim Murphy

This man was kind of a Jekyll-Hyde personality. He had a good side and a bad side that were complete opposites. Most of his bad side came out when he was drinking. This man would sculpt pots for flowers and look after the plants. He sold the plants in order to raise more money for drinking. He was as powerful as a pocket Hulk and used to help people with heavy lifting. He once helped me to lift Mr. Sanchez up some stairs, wheelchair and all. He said, "We should take him over to Canada Packers and sell him."

He was Irish, and some people would say that being Irish accounted for his temper. I have also known many Irish people who do not have bad tempers.

One day, Mr. Murphy came in from an evening of heavy drinking at the bar down the street and started cursing the security guard because it took him a few seconds to answer the door. The security guard called Mr. Martin and told him, "I don't have to take that."

Mr. Martin then called me and said, "Peter, can you tell me what's going on?"

I started saying that I was giving Mr. Watson a bath and . . . Fortunately, a residing supervisor came on the phone at that time and explained what had happened because I did not know until she explained.

Another time, Mr. Murphy came back from a night of heavy drinking and the security guard watching the door was upstairs. This infuriated

Mr. Murphy, so he grabbed the nearest resident and started shaking him viciously. He also started banging tables and chairs and swearing. He then went up to his room to sleep off his drunkenness.

When we went up to see the resident who had been shaken, he was so frightened that he was shaking like a leaf. We were very concerned because this type of action was dangerous. Earlier, he had taken a frail elderly man and dashed him into the ground. He also beat up one of the orderlies. Several times, I had stepped in front of him when he went to attack various residents, and if I had been on hand for this latest incident, it might not have happened. I wrote a detailed report, which Mr. Martin read the next day, and gave him a verbal report that evening as well. Mr. Martin promised drastic action.

The plan was to send Mr. Murphy to a treatment centre for alcoholics that had very pleasant surroundings. Mr. Martin felt that he would like it. When Mr. Murphy refused to go there because he did not want to stop drinking, he was discharged from the home. I saw him selling flowers a few months later and asked him how he was doing. He replied, "I'm growing old gracefully."

He could have been a good resident if we could only have accentuated his positive characteristics and eliminated his negative characteristics. This would not be the last time that I had let someone down by not being there when I was needed.

Mr. Don Mitchell

This man presents a very happy story. He lived to be 104 years old and was strong and active until he was 99. He always went around saying, "I feel as good as I felt when I was fifty."

He did not smoke or drink and watched his diet as carefully as he could. Before he came into the senior citizens' home, he was part vegetarian and only ate meat twice a week. When he came into the home, he had to eat meat every day because that was being served, but he would skip a meal if it was too salty. He had the legs of a football player and prominent biceps as well as rippling muscles. He had only a slight amount of fat on his belly. Until he was ninety-nine, he walked five miles every day. He had worked hard at coal shoveling until he retired at age eighty-four.

Mr. Mitchell did not stop with his physical fitness regimen until age one hundred when he slipped on some ice and broke his hip. He was sent to a hospital where he was not given physiotherapy. This caused the tendons in his leg to shorten so that they were stuck in a bent position, called a "contracture." Because of that, he could not walk anymore and went steadily downhill.

Mr. Mitchell had some interesting ideas on how to take care of himself. In addition to diet and exercise, he believed in the use of lanolin for infections (which is not a good idea). He used Vicks products for many ailments with good results and credits them with saving his life when he had a bout of pneumonia. He was a walking advertisement for Vicks products.

One time, I had to put antibiotics on his toes because he felt he was caring for his toes by pulling his toenails off. Unfortunately, he got an infection. Fortunately, it was resolved.

Mr. Mitchell loved most sports and listened to football, soccer, and hockey games. He himself had played many sports, including lacrosse when he was younger. He could keep a visitor talking for hours about sports. His medical was usually summed up as "very fit for age." Even though he led a long, happy, and healthy life, he will still be missed.

Mr. John Shaw

John Shaw was another resident who did not smoke or drink. He was a very likeable man who endeared himself to many people. In his younger days, he did manual labour on a farm in Ottawa, working fourteen to sixteen hours a day almost every day of the week. He was in good condition at the time, but his epilepsy, decreasing mobility, and lack of balance eventually caught up with him.

One concerned resident stated, "Wherever there's a floor, you don't trust John Shaw," meaning that he would fall whenever he took his eyes off the floor, which happened regularly. We never really found out what went wrong with his balance, but it was probably caused by damage to the balance centre in his brain.

Mr. Shaw had an operation on his elbow to correct numbness in his fingers. The operation helped because it restored nerve transmission from his elbows to his fingers, but the operation left his arm stiff and sore. I did range of motion exercises with him in order to help get rid of the stiffness and, consequently, the pain. After a while, he got better.

In his last two years, Mr. Shaw became incontinent of urine and feces for some reason, and frequently had to be cleaned up. We could not get him cleaned up often enough, because there were so many residents, and as a consequence, he developed skin rashes. Mr. Shaw was always pleasant throughout all his ordeals, and I was sorry to hear of his demise a few years later.

Big Earl Nevills

He stood six foot four weighing 225 lbs, kinda broad at the shoulder, kinda narrow at the hip, and everyone knew you didn't give no lip to Big Earl. After several years of enjoying food, Earl finally put weight on his middle, but he once was a tapered, powerful athlete. In his younger days, he worked at many strenuous manual labour jobs such as coal mining, construction, and ditch digging. He was a veteran of the professional wrestling ring and played football for the Hamilton Tiger-Cats in Canada. He had to work in a steel mill because football did not pay enough at that time. For that matter, neither did professional wrestling. Earl was a military policeman during World War Two. He had a loud, booming voice at times and commanded a great deal of respect. One day, about two weeks after he went to visit his daughter in Columbus, Ohio, I was eagerly awaiting his return. When I was delivering some tea on the third floor, I could hear his voice from the first floor, and I knew that Big Earl was back.

Earl had led a full life in many ways. He had a university education as an engineer and worked at that for a long time. He had several girlfriends and a few wives, the odd one being common-law. He had had a drinking problem early in his life but had overcome it and was very proud of his sobriety. He even came to look down on drinking and said some negative things about alcoholics at times. Earl had overcome a lot of problems in his life, including having a stroke at age forty-nine. It took him several years to recover from this stroke, but he eventually recovered well enough to go back to work. He did not stop working until he had a heart attack that required the insertion of a pacemaker. Unfortunately, he was a heavy smoker and eventually died of complications from chronic obstructive lung disease. With this disease, the air sacs in the lungs break down and there is less area to exchange gases with the blood. Chronic obstructive lung disease puts a strain on the heart because it is difficult to push blood through damaged lungs. This strain can make the heart unable to do its job so that the blood backs up in the jugular vein, the liver, and the tissues. This condition is termed "heart failure."

Getting back to Big Earl and his courage, he had several painful medical problems while at the mission, such as a bowel obstruction, but did not even utter so much as a whimper. Earl was elected president of the resident's council, probably because he was one of the few educated men there. There was a joke question going "Who's the administrator of the senior citizen's home?"

Some people replied, "I thought it was Mr. Nevills."

I often visited Big Earl when I needed a lift, and he would always supply pleasant conversation. I also had to make sure that he was well supplied with Beclovent and Ventolin inhalers, and I tended to keep an eye on him, generally. He needed a lot of care, partly because he needed ointment applied to his foot ulcers. He often found it painful to walk and healed slowly, probably because of his poor circulation. An interesting thing about him is that he got his words mixed up. He called Mr. Westergaard, "Mr. Overgaard," and Valisone-G was "valen G." I later learned that this was probably from his old stroke.

Earl lived to be seventy-six, surviving several scrapes. At one point, his lungs were so bad that only two areas the size of a woman's fists were working. That was successfully treated, but I always worried about him. He was one of the finest men that I have met, and I wish I could see him again.

Mr. Jim Parsons

Here was an interesting man. He was very tough and unselfish. He once said, "I hope things get better for the younger people of this country. Things were not very good for me, but I have had my shot at life."

Mr. Parsons suffered from rheumatoid arthritis that became very painful in his last few years. He said that sometimes all he could do for the pain was get drunk. He had nodes and deformities on many of his joints. He used to like to watch wrestling at Maple Leaf Gardens and have a few beers while he was out. He would come back for large dosages of antacids to get rid of the sore stomach caused by the beers.

Here was a man who had been a lumberjack all his life and worked despite great pain. He was one of the persons whom skid row was named after, as I mentioned earlier. He was usually good-natured and joking, but when his arthritis got bad, he became very cantankerous. He ended up suffering a heart attack and getting over it. He lost about one hundred pounds when his arthritis got bad, and he did not feel like eating.

He became very sour on everyone, due mostly to his pain, and one day, he left for Sudbury up north to get away from all the "bad people." He ended up dying of a fatal heart attack there, and if I knew him, he probably refused help from anyone. He was a good friend most of the time and told me that I took good care of him. He cared about the other residents and urged the man on duty to do something about his roommate, Mr. Shubert, who was unusually restless. The man who was on duty—who was on loan from an agency—did nothing, and Mr. Shubert died probably of congestive heart failure and pulmonary edema. I let Mr. Shubert down because if I had been there that night, he might not have died.

Joe Shubert

This was an interesting man. He was a very heavy drinker and justified his drinking as a cure for his dizziness. He had a disease called Meniere's disease, which is an ear infection that damages balance and hearing. Both these functions are partially controlled by the ear. Joe's disease did not bother him too much and would mostly flare up when he was drinking. Mr. Shubert's explanation was that his ear was blocked, and it made his brain turn around. He said that he was willing to try anything for a cure, so he drank Canadian sherry. Joe was deaf most of the time but had particular difficulty hearing when you told him something he did not want to hear, like "it's time for your bath." I could usually get through to him by writing notes or talking loudly.

Joe eventually developed hepatitis from drinking. His eyeballs turned yellow, and he developed a stomach bleed from drinking too much. The bleeding stomach caused his hemoglobin, which is the part of the blood that transports oxygen, to drop dramatically. This can cause dilation of the blood vessels to compensate for the decreased ability of the blood to transport oxygen. The dilated blood vessels, in turn, can overload the heart and cause heart failure. Heart failure, in turn, can cause the lungs to fill up with fluid and damage breathing. I was not present for Mr. Shubert's death, but my guess is that he died from his lungs filling up with fluid. He was a good friend and never caused any trouble, drunk or sober.

Mr. Shubert, I should mention, suffered from "the heartbreak of psoriasis." He had smelly sores all over his body, but as long as we put cortisone on his sores, they were very mild. They would only start to look angry if he missed a cortisone treatment. As an illustration of how little some men care about themselves, we left the cortisone by his bedside and he never used it.

Myths and Truths About Alcoholism

One statement made about drinking problems is that in order to quit, one must stop drinking entirely. I found that with the men in the home, they fell into a number of groups. One group would drink at every opportunity. These men were not motivated at all to quit. However, few of them would show signs of missing alcohol if they could not get it. They just carried on their normal lives. Another group would stop for the most part and only occasionally lose control and get drunk. I did find that very few of the men in the home were social drinkers. Once they took a drink, they would tend to get drunk.

Another statement about drinking is that after achieving sobriety, alcoholics lose their craving for alcohol. I found that this was true for the most part, especially when the men were proud of their sobriety. Earl Nevills never touched a drop of alcohol after stopping and deeply resented being referred to as an alcoholic.

Another statement about alcoholism is that alcoholics cannot stop after their first drink. I found that this was true for the most part.

Another statement about alcoholics is that they have more problems than nondrinkers. I did not find this to be true for the most part. The drinkers in the home were not much different from the sober men.

It has been said about alcoholics that they tend to separate themselves from family and friends. I found that the men in the home had few visitors and tended to be loners, except when they were actively drinking.

Another statement about alcoholism is that alcoholics are embarrassing and difficult. This was true about some of the alcoholics in the home. In some men, alcohol drew out the worst in them, but most of the men were likeable, even when drunk.

It has also been stated about alcoholism that alcoholics feel self-hatred and hatred of those around them. This is too extreme a statement. The men in the home tended not to care about themselves when they drank, but they cared about themselves when they were sober. They also tended to get rough with others when they drank, but this did not amount to actual hatred. There was sometimes a one-time tendency to mild violence, like punching someone, but it went away once they sobered up.

A myth about alcoholism is that secret drinking distinguishes alcoholics. Most of the men in the home made no attempt to drink secretly.

One thing that I found to be true about alcoholics is that they tend to encourage others to drink. They often like company and like to share the drinking experience. Some of the men would even offer me a drink, which I always declined. They may have encouraged others to drink to decrease their own guilt about drinking.

Another myth about skid row is that it is the rundown section of town where bums and winos live and drink together. As I explained earlier, this is just not true. There are probably as many alcoholics among middle-class and wealthy people as among poor people. Some of the men in the home started out very wealthy, even millionaires, but drank up most of their money. Others could not hold down a job because of drinking problems, but this was not always the case.

The main things that I attempted to do in my work in the whole field was to work for the benefit of the patients, care about them, and encourage them to care about themselves. I had varying degrees of success, but caring itself is a therapeutic process and a little bit can go a long way.

The point that I want to make is that alcoholics are likeable, even loveable, people. There is a very wealthy woman that I know who is also beautiful, sexy, intelligent, kind, warm, loving, affectionate, and courageous. I frequently help her when she goes into delirium tremens, which is a withdrawal from alcoholic binging. She shakes uncontrollably and has several anxiety attacks caused by the discharge of nerve cells that are used to getting their alcohol to depress them. She is an example of how outandly likeable an alcoholic can be.

I found that when Becky went into delirium tremens, she felt better when she was touched and cuddled. Our bodies are vehicles of healing.

The Twelve Steps of Alcoholics Anonymous

1. We must admit that we are powerless over alcohol, that our lives have become unmanageable.
2. Come to believe that a power greater than ourselves could restore us to sanity.
3. Make a decision to turn our will and our lives over to the care of God as we understand him.
4. Make a searching and fearless moral inventory of ourselves.
5. Admit to all the nature of our wrongs.
6. Let God remove the flaws of our character.
7. Humbly ask him to remove our shortcomings.
8. Make a list of all people we've harmed and try to make amends with them.
9. Try to make amends with people we have harmed, except when it would cause more harm.
10. Admit when we are wrong.
11. Pray to God and find his plan.
12. Having had a spiritual awakening as a result of these steps, we should try to carry this message to others and continue to practice the principles in all our affairs.

Rational-Emotive Therapy of Alcoholism

Rational-emotive therapy consists of getting rid of irrational thinking. First, we have A, the activating event, then B, the belief system (rational or irrational). C is the consequence; in this case, drinking. D is to dispute the irrational belief. Irrational beliefs consist of shoulds, oughts, and musts that just are not true and perpetuate the problem. If someone treats you badly, an alcoholic would say, "I must have drink to feel better." He must dispute this belief and realize that the world has good and bad people in it, and we must cope with both.

It has been my finding that different people drink for different reasons. The similarity is in the way that they handle the problem. The irrational belief in alcoholism is that one must drink. The patient must use D and dispute the irrational belief.

Chrissy's Song

This is the story of a courageous woman who made many never-ending successes and suffered some agonizing defeats. Among her successes were making the Ontario scholarship roll and getting straight A's in university. She was also described by a friend as a wonderful mother. She still has not conquered smoking and drinking but has made great inroads.

This girl first noticed that something was wrong with her family when she noticed that her father was less affectionate toward her mother. She asked her mother if she and Daddy were going to separate, and her mother said no. Her father also threw plates at the wall and got a divorce when Miss C was only eight. She said that it was very hurtful. Her father said that his girlfriend gave a better blow job than his wife and took off. He was financially supportive and very wealthy but was not emotionally supportive. When Miss C was eight, she would cry, cry, and cry.

Miss C's mother was depressed. When a child loses a parent at a young age, it can do lasting damage—which later may have resulted in Miss C's problems. She developed bulimia nervosa to satisfy her parents that she be thin. She felt that she must earn her parents' love and tended to blame herself for her parents' divorce.

How We Met

I first met Miss C during a time when a fire took away the power to our building. I noticed that she was cute and innocent-looking. I offered to take her to dinner because she could not cook.

We went to the only restaurant that was open. I was puzzled because she ordered two tall glasses of wine and finally some mussels. I thought she would order something essential. It wasn't until later that I realized she had a drinking problem. Also, I did not know how beautiful and sexy she could be when she wanted.

She had two of the most beautiful and exciting breasts that she brazenly exposed in order to have a back massage. Sometimes, her nipples would be hard and swollen, which was even more exciting. She said that there was nothing wrong with showing the human body but had trouble understanding how exciting she was.

I also found her friendly and affectionate, which is also a virtue. She always sold herself short. She was a wonderful mother, as one of her friends confirmed.

One of her favorite songs, which she said described her, went: "I'm a bitch, I'm a lover, I'm a child, I'm a mother." I never felt that she was cruel so that anything negative about her being a "bitch" was not deserved. She had a heart of gold, which she showed in countless ways.

One time she invited a homeless man to stay in her apartment. The man was homeless because he had schizophrenia and was impotent from his medication.

Miss C had a tendency to attract abusive men because she was borderline for a masochistic personality disorder, which was diagnosed by her psychologists. She looked for love in all the wrong places. I also felt that she was overly casual about sex. She did not have poor morals but did not believe in getting to know someone before she had sex with him. In spite of that, her relationships with men were always faithful, as far as I know.

Miss C found that her father was never there for her and was always having affairs. Her mother could not help her much either because she was overwhelmed by her own depression regarding her divorce. Her father ran off with her mother's best friend.

Miss C was also upset about her father not letting her see one of her stepmothers, with whom she had a good rapport.

She felt embarrassed to bring friends over. Her mother and sister were always fighting, so her mother sent her sister to her father in Nassau. Her father kicked her out at age sixteen. She then went to live with her boyfriend.

Miss C feels that her life is like a soap opera. If you read on, you will find out why.

When Miss C was eight, she had some best friends, whom she referred to as needs. One day, she got into a fight with Greek girls because they called her friend and her names. They ran off and were free.

At age fifteen, Miss C developed bulimia. Her mother was not there, and she lost fifteen pounds.

Her first boyfriend was a guy named Jason. He called her Porky, which aggravated her eating disorder. He was verbally abusive. Miss C had a pattern of having abusive relationships, and one of the men almost killed her.

Miss C lost her virginity to Jason one month before she turned eighteen. She was ninety-four pounds and wanted to disappear. She felt unworthy because of her father's leaving.

Throughout the interview, Miss C was crying because she felt the story was very sad. Kelly did not want to acknowledge her abuse, and Miss C expected the abuse.

However, Miss C felt that Jason treated her well. She had her first French kiss with him. It felt strange, according to her. When she lost her virginity, she bled from a ruptured hymen. It sounded kind of sad.

Miss C's stepmom was sweet and nice. She left her father because he cheated too often. She fought with Mr. C. Miss C went to visit her father but was arrested for stealing his car. She was released when they found out that it wasn't her who took the car.

When Miss C was nineteen, she got a scholarship to go to the University of Toronto and decided on Western University. She finished her high school in Switzerland and went from 140 pounds to 120. She got rid of most of her bulimia there.

Miss C did very well at Western and got her BA in psychology. She took nutrition at Ryerson so that she could help others with eating disorders. She got pregnant on her third year. She was twenty-seven at the time and did not want to make a life with her baby's father. She looked after the baby for four years and was a wonderful mother. When Miss C started to have emotional problems, the father took charge of the baby.

Miss C's parents gave her material things but did not give her much time or emotional support.

When Miss C could not locate her daughter, she had a major anxiety attack. Her partner was so overweight that he could hardly walk, but eventually, she found her daughter.

Miss C said that you could write a dream if you are really passionate. Miss C's story is certainly passionate. When Miss C had her daughter, she had postpartum depression but still carried on as an excellent mother.

Miss C has been in a number of rehabilitation centers for alcoholism. So far, there has been no lasting result. One of the times that she went to a rehabilitation center was after her boyfriend beat her up and broke several bones, including her tailbone. She was at Bellwoods, Austen Riggs, and a few others. She found the staff insensitive, especially when they did nothing to help a suicidal girl. She also found the psychiatrist to be a nightmare who had no respect for her.

In university, Miss C was an excellent student. However, she looked for love in all the wrong places. Bulimia and sexual obsession tend to go together; Miss C's bulimia started when she was thirteen.

When Miss C was twenty-three and twenty-four, she took a trip around the world, starting at Toronto. She overcame her eating disorder and gained twenty pounds.

What the Experts Say

One psychologist said that Miss C's parents' divorce when she was eight years old was extremely important. Miss C says that she drinks to get away from bad memories. Miss C noticed that her parents were not getting along well and that her father was less affectionate toward her mother.

She did not like the job. She was lonely, resumed drinking, and occasionally was bulimic. In November, she took a mild overdose of something and was taken to the Clarke Institute of Psychiatry.

Around the time that she seemed to have resolved to turn her life around and get on top of her problems, she met her fiancé, Todd number 2. She considered him a godsend: open, honest, down-to-earth, and great with children. He was an actor and enjoyed acting. Together, they started a film production company. Todd was nine and a half years younger than Miss C.

Miss C had turned herself and learned a number of coping skills at the Addiction Research Foundation. She does not need medication, except for the occasional Valium every four months or so.

Most of Miss C's IQ scores were above average, but some were decreased because of anxiety.

Her affinity to alcohol might partly represent a means of filling the emptiness of life, the anxiety reduction, anger, confusion, and to solve depression. Alcohol is an abusive partner that is less than human—a drug. She may have had some sexual abuse that taught her to seek out abusive partners.

Miss C may have had a number of vulnerabilities that put her off track, but she is trying to get on track again. She seemed to be someone who has suffered and struggled considerably and who sometimes embraced maladaptive pseudosolutions to her problems. She seems to have developed emotional coping skills that will stand her in good stead as she proceeds.

Assessments showed that Miss C is fully capable of caring for her daughter on weekends without supervision.

Miss C's urine came up negative for alcohol 95 percent of the time in the year 2000 to 2001.

Miss C's diagnostic impression from a therapist at Austen Riggs Treatment Centre follows: "Dysthymic or mood disorder, eating disorder, bulimia nervosa, in which she spits out her food; alcohol dependence, borderline personality disorder, coccygeal fracture from boyfriend, problems in relation to family of origin, relationships with others, and caring for her daughter."

Miss C worries about the danger of her rage about being abandoned. She acts out her overwhelming dependent longings and rage with significant others, although I have never seen her angry.

Miss C has been involved with a number of men who have been controlling and abusive. These relationships may, in various ways, remind her of her relationship with her father.

My Experience With Barbara

I am writing this to describe my experience with a prostitute to give much-needed insight into prostitution and also human nature. There may be many misconceptions among people about prostitutes and about human sexuality in general. I do not say that this one experience will necessarily give any definitive knowledge, but I do feel that it gives some insight into prostitution and sexuality. I also feel that I cannot speak for all prostitutes. There may be some that do not fit my description at all. I have never endeavored to get to know an active prostitute as well as Barbara due to this bad experience, but I suspect that there are more prostitutes like her.

A study of prostitutes by James and Meyerding[1], who compared the histories of prostitutes with "normal" women, found that prostitutes differed significantly in that they:

1. learned less about sex from their parents and more from personal experience.
2. as children, experienced more sexual advances by elders.
3. were more often involved in incestuous relationships with their fathers.
4. more often had no further relationship with their first coital partner.
5. generally initiated sexual activity at a younger age.
6. experienced a higher incidence of rape and violence.

Let us see if my story bears this out. Although this story reads like a fiction story, it is totally true and nonfictional.

It started when I decided that I wanted my first sexual experience. Up until then, I believed that premarital sex was wrong. However, as I started to get older, I became depressed because I wanted more contact with women and also sexual contact. I worried that I would become impotent before I had had my first experience. I wanted sex to have the pleasure of giving a woman pleasure and to help me relate to women. I decided on the escort services in the yellow pages as the avenue to explore. I did this because I felt that it would cause the girls the least damage because these girls would be having sex often anyway, and they would be protected from pregnancy. It bothered my conscience a little, but I very much wanted the experience. I suspected that most of the escort services were prostitutes because of the suggestive ads, the sexy recording over the phone, and the tremendous amount of money that they charged for only one hour's visit (between $150 and $300). I settled on an agency called First Time because I felt that it would be the most appropriate and the girl would be understanding. I later found out that they were only interested in making money and did not care about helping anyone with a first time. Indeed, the girl did not believe that it was my first time anyway. First Time Escorts has since gone out of business.

I called them up, and a woman answered the phone: "First Time." I asked about having a girl. She told me to get a hotel room, and she would get a girl to call me. I told her that I did not want to pay for a hotel room, and she replied, "I know someone who is willing to entertain in her own home. I will have her call."

A few minutes later, the phone rang, and a girl spoke and told me that her name was Rena and that she would be my girl. I later found out that the girl, Rena, and the girl that answered the phone were really one and the same, and she was disguising her voice so that I would not know that they were the same person. I also later found out that this girl ran the agency with her pimp and that they shared the profits. She did the booking of clients, the bookkeeping, and kept files on the clients so that they knew who was "weird" or unpleasant and who did not pay, etc. This girl also went out on most of the calls. This girl also later told me that her real name was not Rena and that she kept a different name for each client.

At any rate, she told me that there would be a $40 agency fee and $200 for the "tip." She described herself and attractiveness and told me how to get to her place. I felt a bit of guilt and a bit of nervousness, but this was greatly overshadowed by my determination to have my first sexual experience. I wondered what it would be like and if I could actually do it. I also felt a pleasant sexual excitement about going to this girl.

I got to her apartment and rang her code number. A few seconds later, an attractive woman came out wearing high heels and a skimpy exercise suit. She invited me in and told me to sit down on her couch. She talked to me and gave me some apple juice. She asked me what I did and talked about herself a little, all in an effort to relax me. I did not tell her that it was my first time. She told how she left the army because she wanted to run this business and was afraid that the army would dishonourably discharge her if they found out about the business. I found this to be strange because I could not understand why she would need the business if she had a good job in the army. From my later experience with her, I developed an idea that prostitution is a type of compulsive disease that women practice for various reasons. She came over to me and sat beside me. I put my hand on her leg and began to wonder if she would really give me sex because she seemed totally disinterested and maybe a little repulsed by my touch. I asked if she was married because I did not want to have sex with a married woman. She said that she was divorced and had one son. Her son was outside playing so that he would not see us together. I paid her, and we moved into the bedroom.

The sex was great. She took down the strap to her exercise suit and noticed that I didn't have an erection.

"What's the matter?" she asked.

I told her that I was on some medication and needed some time. I lay down on the floor and asked, "Can I look at you? You are very beautiful."

"Thank you." She said

I stared at her beautiful, full, lanky body with my eyes coming to rest on her gorgeous breasts. They looked like pear-shaped balloons, only fuller, and I later found out later just that they were as good to feel as to look at. When she saw that I had an erection, she rushed over to me, applied a condom, and guided me into her.

She began to thrust with her hips, which got me even more excited. At that point, I lost my fear of not getting an erection and got caught up in the pleasure of the moment.

She said that having sex is like playing with yourself, that you need a massaging motion in order to ejaculate. I began to thrust up and down myself in intense delight.

Incredibly, she then crushed her mouth mercilessly down on mine as she lay on top of me. It was so exciting, so sensual, that I would remember it for a long, long time. Her lips were like wine with an electric sensuality about them. After a few more thrusts, she asked, "Did you come yet?"

I answered, "No, it would probably take me a long time."

We rolled over, kissed again, and I could feel her vagina getting wetter.

"Do you enjoy this?" I asked.

"Sometimes," she answered. "This time, I do."

I reached my hand up to touch her breast and felt her flesh like a balloon that had just been blown up and was soft, yet firm, and as delicious as vanilla ice cream. It was the first time I had ever touched a full-grown woman's bare breast. It was wonderfully exciting. We kept on thrusting and massaging each other as well as hugging each other as if we had been friends for a long time and not as if we had just met.

We changed positions several times, and finally, when she was on top, she began to thrust viciously.

"Could you stop thrusting?" I asked.

"I can't, I've got ants in my pants!" she answered.

I started to laugh with joy. I wondered why I had missed an experience like this for so long. I was definitely ready for it.

She asked, "Why are you laughing?"

I replied, "I'm very happy."

"Thank you," she replied.

"I feel like I could lie here for two days straight," she moaned.

Finally, we lay together, content, with her body at first back on top of me and then we lay side by side. The session was supposed to last an hour or less, but we ended up making love for an hour and a half. She raised up her tall, lanky, naked body like a goddess of love who had just tended to someone's needs, her skin taking on the golden colour of her hair, her breasts and thick thighs bouncing sexily.

I told her, "This is my first time."

"Get out of here, this isn't your first time. I could tell by your hip motion."

"Yes, it was my first time," I answered.

"You should have told me it was your first time," she said.

She reached her hand out and touched my belly.

"It's hard as a rock," she said. "Maybe that's where you've been all this time."

I once again touched her soft belly and said, "You have an impressive femininity.

"Thank you," she said.

For six weeks after that, I remained on a lover's high and got an erection every time I thought about her.

She later went to pick up her son. Before she left, I felt so elated with the experience and so fond of her that I kissed her all over her face and hugged her. She was indifferent to my affection. She got her son, and I said good-bye to her and her son. She told her son, "Say good-bye to the nice man, Danny." Danny waved, and I was off.

I felt elated and fond of her for the next several weeks. I wondered why she had become a prostitute. I thought that maybe if I showed her a little love and affection that I could change her from being a prostitute. I felt that I sort of loved her. I called her one night a few weeks later and told her how much I enjoyed the experience and enjoyed being with her and asked if I could see her socially. She asked, "What's the matter? Are you lonely?" I said no. I left it at that and told that I would call back when I wanted to see her professionally again. Reflecting back on when we had sex, I had asked her if she enjoyed sex. She said, "Sometimes." She was indifferent to my play all through the experience, reluctant to be fondled or caressed, and was being mechanical in her kisses and hip thrusting, always wishing that I would finish and get it over with.

A few weeks later, I called and wanted to see her the next day. She told me to meet her at a hotel because she had changed apartments and could not see me at her apartment. I had two weeks' vacation coming up, and I thought it would be a good time to see her. When I saw her, I brought some flowers for her. She said that she was sick and did not feel up to sex, so I took her out to lunch. We talked about several things, and I found that she was very intelligent despite having no formal education. She was teaching herself grade 1 biology and chemistry. She talked about how she had a history of pelvic inflammatory disease and felt that she might be having another bout of it. I told her that I would look up information on pelvic inflammatory disease in my nursing textbook of obstetrics and read it to her. The symptoms that she described could have been peritonitis.

The next day, I made a long two-hour trip to the hospital, bringing a radio and some of my favorite books, all of which she has never returned. When I got there, I was relieved to find out that she was not really as sick as she described. The pain was not too bad, and she could walk. She said, "I feel rotten, but I'm glad you're here." I went over to her and kissed her and hugged her. I held her hand for a while and then got her some food. She had also marked off every food item on her menu, which had to be corrected because she would have been eating too much. She was rude with the head nurse about this. This was the first time I had noticed rudeness in her. We held hands and talked for a few hours, and I was about to go home.

She asked, "Do you have any money?"

I asked, "What for?"

She said, "For food for my son."

Concerned about her family, I gave some of the money that I had. Over the next few days, I continued to help her financially. She remained aloof but friendly to an extent. She did not force me to maintain contact with her or give her money, but she did not discourage it. She once seemed to laugh at what a "stupid idiot" I was for getting into a car accident. I still wonder if she really had contempt for me.

All this time, she declined to let me visit her place, giving numerous excuses. Finally, she let me visit her apartment. That night—taking her home from the hospital to her apartment—I got to sit with her son, her, and two babysitters. After an hour or two, she told me what was going on with her. She told me that she had been harassed at her old apartment, so she latched on to a customer who told her that he would live with her in a new apartment and support her and her son. It later turned out that this customer had no money and could not keep up rent on her apartment or support her. He really wanted to live off her. He was also violent and bad-tempered. He hit her son and smashed her stereo and frequently threatened her with a knife. She showed me a hole in the wall where this man had put his fist through the wall. She asked me if I would help her move so we could get an apartment together. I told her that since I was so fond of her, that I would help her move and wanted to see her out of this bad situation.

On my way home, I got some newspapers to look for a new place for her to live. Over the next few days, I helped her move her belongings into a moving van, which I rented, and babysat with her son while she looked for a new apartment. The man that she had been living with had been thrown out of the apartment by the police and was only allowed back to the apartment to get his belongings. Helping us move was a man named Jack, who she said was her ex-boyfriend. For the first time, Barbara seemed to get short-tempered easily and also started to swear profusely, which I had never heard her do before. She also had no interest in any sex or affection and seemed to be repulsed by any touching. When I mentioned this aspect of her personality to her, she said that she was not herself because of all the stress that she had been going through. I asked if there was any chance that we could become friends. She answered, "You're a very good friend, look at all the things you do for me." All along, I had hoped that she would become a friend, but the relationship was all give on my part and none on hers. I had also hoped that I could change her, but to no avail.

It turned out that Frank, the man that she had been living with, was even more dangerous than we thought. He caught us moving and demanded that Barbara give him the keys to the apartment, or he would hit her. I stepped in front of him and told him to leave. Barbara threatened to call the police, and he backed off and went back to his car. He said that he would get back at us and drove off. He later came back with a friend but left when he saw that Jack and I were there. I knew while I was sitting in the apartment with Barbara's son that he would be back.

One day, while sitting in the apartment with Danny, Barbara's son, there was a knock at the door. Frank said, "Let us in." I recognized Frank's voice and saw two men through the peephole. I felt that I would not be able to handle two men and that they would pose a threat to Danny and me. I kept the door locked and said that I was just waiting; they could return at any time. Danny had wanted to unlock the door when they came and frequently wanted to unlock the door. Although he was very likeable, he was very difficult to manage and did not understand what was going on, thinking it was all a game. He played many games with me, frequently ordering me around, and he could not sit still or be quiet. He did not understand the need for quiet or my need for rest. Later, when we were finishing the move, we dumped Frank's belongings into the hall for him to pick up. A gun and several bullets fell out of Frank's briefcase. We called the police and showed them the gun and bullets. They said that they would investigate the matter further. I do not know what became of Frank, but I was glad when Barbara found a place to live and we could finish moving. I knew that Frank was a very dangerous man. On a cold fall night, I helped Barbara move into her new place.

At this time, Barbara was going through some legal trouble of her own. She had run up a large bill on one of her ex-boyfriends' credit cards and was facing charges for fraud for which she had to appear in court. She said that she had been used and abused by this man and felt that she had the right to run up a bill on his credit card because he had given it to her for that purpose. The only reason that he had pressed charges, according to her, was because she refused to live with him. It turned out that after her court appearance, she was given a one-thousand-dollar fine for fraud. If she did not pay it by 5 p.m. that day, she would face six months in jail. She told me that her grandfather had wired in one thousand dollars to pay the fine, but she could not get it in time to pay by 5 p.m. and asked if I would pay the fine and be reimbursed. I did not want her to go to jail, so I agreed and we went off to withdraw the money from my bank and pay the fine.

After we paid the fine, I took Barbara and Danny to dinner. I had an uneasy feeling all that day that she would not pay back the money that I loaned her, and had difficulty eating because of this feeling. Later that night, I helped Barbara finish moving. I bought her some clothes so that she would not be cold while we were moving. I lifted the very heavy furniture that she was not able to lift. Barbara left me in the new apartment to guard the furniture while she cleaned up the old apartment. When she did not come back after two hours, I got the distinct feeling that she had tricked me and was not coming back at all. I called the old apartment several times with no result. After another hour of that, I felt sure that she had left me and I went home. I felt tricked, cheated, deceived, and devastated. It turned out that I was wrong about her not coming back but was not wrong about being cheated.

The next morning, I was very upset because I was lost without any money, having loaned her most of my life's savings. My sister needed a loan, and I could only give her the small remnants of my life's savings. My brother-in-law was a lawyer who told me that I had trusted her too much and so had not left a legal outlet to get the money back. That morning, Barbara called and told me that she had been worried about me all night and could not sleep. She explained that she had taken a long time cleaning up the old apartment before going to the new apartment. I told her that I felt that she had tricked me. She told me that she fully intended to pay the money back. However, when I asked her to come down to Union Station with me to get the money that her grandfather had sent, she said that she was busy moving. When I said that I wanted to help her move and then get the money, she said, "No, don't worry about it, I want to do it myself." She pretended to sympathize with how upset I was and told me that if I wanted to call to ventilate my feelings that I could leave a message with the babysitter. I frantically tried to reach her apartment but I could not remember where it was, and there was a snowstorm that slowed the buses. I also knew that I had very little money left and would have to work hard to earn back what I had lost. After several attempts to find her apartment, I ran into the streets and started screaming. Fortunately, the cars did not hit me and went around me. I knew that I was suicidal and needed help. When I got home, I phoned my family doctor. He told me to go to the nearest hospital for help. At the hospital, I got enough help so that I was no longer suicidal and was able to carry on again. I left very encouraged and no longer needing help. I started exercising and studying and keeping busy. I resolved that I would start dating again after I had earned back some money.

Barbara was not doing very well. She became bedridden with mononucleosis and a bloated belly, which took months for the doctors to diagnose as ovarian cysts. She could not look after her son and needed care herself. Over the next few weeks, I helped her with groceries, housework, babysitting for Danny, and with using my nursing skills and knowledge to help her. I got to know her much better. Although she was dishonest with me in many ways, she was also honest with me in many ways. She tried to cheat me out of money many times, but I would only buy the minimum groceries necessary and would not fall for her stories. Buying her groceries slowed my earning back the money that I had lost, but I was working harder than ever, and with much overtime, I was earning more than usual. Eventually, after a few weeks, I decided that I did not owe her anything and should not carry the burden of supporting her, so I called several social service agencies and finally found one that would take over for me with nursing help and financial help and babysitting.

Barbara eventually got better several weeks later and called me to tell me that she was better. She told me that the money that her grandfather had given her was stolen, but that she was earning money again (she did not say how) and that she would pay me back eventually. After that, I did not hear from her for several weeks. At the time that I heard from her several weeks later, she was in legal and financial trouble again and was sick again with an illness that I never found out more about. She had just gotten out of jail for something that she said was not her fault and described several family members dying and several troubles that she had gone through. She asked if I could come to visit her. "Oh, I'm so sorry." I suspected that she wanted to cheat me out of more money and told her that I did not want to visit her if that was the case. She told me, "When you decide that I am harmless, come and visit." That was the last that I heard from her. The next day, she was discharged from the hospital and I had no way of contacting her. Two years later, I have still not heard from her, and her family has moved away.

In the weeks that I was looking after Barbara, she told me much about her life and experiences. When she was young, her parents often beat her and strongly believed in physical punishment. She also used physical punishment on her son, even though she loved him dearly. When Barbara was nine, her father raped her. Shortly after that, her parents separated. Her mother bore resentment towards her and blamed her for the husband leaving. She frequently said, "Why don't you go be a hooker on Yonge St.?" She kept her around the house and would not let her date or try to develop a career in spite of the fact that she had many talents and interests. Her mother encouraged the other children to hit her and abuse her. When Barbara was fifteen, her mother threw her out of the house along with a few possessions. She divided up most of Barbara's possessions among the other children. She told Barbara to go away and be a hooker on Yonge St.

Barbara became a ward of the Children's Aid Society. The CAS would not let her work, which she wanted, so she went to live with a Greek immigrant at age fifteen and went to work. The Greek immigrant did not work, so Barbara supported him. He drank up a good part of the money and confiscated it so that Barbara could not go anywhere. At nineteen, Barbara and the man got married. A year later, they had a son.

All this time, Barbara remained faithful to him. A few months after the birth of the son, the husband started to beat Barbara. One time, it took a long recuperation for her to recover. Barbara soon got a divorce. Her husband's sister looked after the son while she was sick. Barbara was very depressed after the divorce and made two suicide attempts, both times coming very close to death. She also had many bills to pay but that she had to be a devoted mother in spite of many faults and gave much love, attention, affection, and effort to the care of her son. She always put his welfare above anything, with the exception of her compulsion to make money by foul or fair means. She made sure that she gave Danny the best of entertainment, such as trick or treating on Halloween, and made sure that he ate well and generally considered his well-being important.

After her divorce, she decided to become a prostitute for several reasons. She said that she liked the excitement of meeting men, needed the money, and liked the excitement of being a prostitute. She found many boyfriends from her work, most of whom she used much to their disadvantage. One of her boyfriends, whom she met through her work, was the man Jack who had helped us move and had helped Barbara move. Together, they started up their escort services: First Time and Hollywood. Jack became the owner and lived off it. This made him a pimp, although Barbara would not use that word. Jack had a wife and family and got part of the money from the escort service. However, while the service was doing well, he always treated Barbara well and shared money with her. Barbara was an equal partner and hoped to someday become rich from the escort service. However, when the newspapers stopped accepting ads from escort services, the business went downhill and eventually went bankrupt. The pimp, Jack, was very protective of Barbara and threatened to beat up anyone who mistreated her. He also helped look after her when she was sick. However, eventually, he did not come to see her for several weeks while she was sick. At this time, Barbara wanted to start up some legitimate business ventures. Jack was one of the few men Barbara did not take advantage of.

Barbara told me that when someone, a customer, was nice to her, she would be nice to him and they got along well. That explained why she was nice to me as a customer. She viewed her job as giving a man an orgasm and getting paid for it. However, she admitted that she did not like to give or receive pleasure on the job and felt that sex should go along with caring. She did not like men who chased after her for sex and tended to give in only to use them and get things from them. Her main ambition in life was to make a better life for herself and her son. She wanted to become wealthy. She wanted to give up prostitution because she had some bad experiences with violent men and because she disliked the legal troubles that she tended to encounter. Sometimes, I would see her very upset about being caught between a desire to make money and a desire to lead a happy life free from the hounding of legal troubles and the hounding of conscience. One time when she was upset before having to appear before the police for her probation ritual, we hugged and caressed each other (briefly). This was one of the few times that Barbara showed affection. This showed that she had it in her. Also, she told me of how she used to support foster children for the Children's Aid Society. She liked children and had potential for good.

Barbara had few people that she could turn to for guidance, except for her probation officer. Unfortunately, she seemed to have too much contempt for me, for some strange reason, to use me for counseling. I could have helped her much more if she had listened to me and been more honest with me. I hope that someday Barbara can use some of her potential for good and bring out her good qualities to make a better life for herself and her son.

I have drawn several hypotheses about human nature, sexuality, and prostitution from this experience.

About human nature:

Man's mating drive is different from that of some other animals. Some other animals just want to have intercourse. Man has a desire to develop a close relationship with the opposite sex. I could have had pure sex more easily by keeping my relationship with Barbara more businesslike. Instead, I tried to develop a close relationship. This is one reason why sex among humans is better when a close relationship is established first (there are other reasons). When I found an honest woman a few months later, it was easier not to give in to Barbara.

Here are my hypotheses about prostitution:

1. It is a totally useless occupation because the only thing that a prostitute accomplishes is to cheat men out of money. The sexual experience is focused mostly on money, with only a small amount on affection and pleasure and only in some cases. Sex without affection, just for physical release, is pointless and accomplishes nothing. It does not even teach sexual competence because there is no interest in sharing pleasure. Also, the concept of sexual competence is a childish attitude. In a good relationship, there is no concept of performance, only sharing.

2.   Alex Comfort[2], in his book *The Joy of Sex*, said that the most common reason for a woman becoming a prostitute is a hatred of men. My experience with Barbara seemed to back this up. A feminist group wanted to have only the customers of prostitutes charged and not the prostitutes themselves, saying that prostitutes are being exploited by men. This is like charging the victims of thieves but not the thieves themselves. The most common reason for men using prostitutes is lack of sexual contact with women. This is just a biological drive, not the fault of women or men. However, think seriously whether prostitutes are worth the trouble. There may be a small amount of merit in the complaint that prostitutes' clients use them. However, prostitutes use their clients much more and in a much more sinister way, charging them for something that should not be done for money.

3.   We see by Barbara's unpleasant past that there is much merit to the claims by James and Meyerding at the beginning of the article about prostitutes having a violent past with rape, incest, assault, and an unhappy family life. This may be what causes some women to hate men and become prostitutes. However, I feel that ultimately the choice of one's lifestyle belongs to the individual and is the individual's responsibility. I do not feel that there is sufficient excuse for prostitution in our welfare state, with all our social programs.

4.   If a prostitute is to be rehabilitated, she must want help, and one must be firm with her lying and cheating. All my love did not help Barbara as far as I know. I knew a girl who had been rehabilitated from prostitution and turned out to lead a very good life. Prostitutes can be rehabilitated and should not have it held against them, but do not do it at your expense.

5.   Prostitution is a type of mental disease. We saw how Barbara had the potential for much kindness. She was a devoted mother. She was generous to children and to certain friends and had many good qualities and did some good things. Yet with several men, including myself, she was vicious. I was very good to her, yet she almost killed me on more than one occasion. I suspect that Barbara left a good job in the army and the chance at several good careers because prostitution filled several needs:

     (a)   A need for affection.
     (b)   A need to get back at men by cheating them.

(c)   A desire for a great deal of money with little work.
(e)   A desire for male companionship.
(f)   A desire for excitement.

In rehabilitating prostitutes, we need to eliminate some of the causes. Some prostitutes are easier to rehabilitate than others, depending on their reasons for turning to prostitution. One must develop a caring, nurturing rapport with them and teach them to satisfy their needs—financial, emotional, etc.—in a responsible way. I felt that it was important to share my experience and share a story that has not been told in quite the same way.

Footnotes

Comfort, A. The Joy of Sex. Simon and Schuster publishing. New York, New York, 1972.
Mims, F. and Swenson, M. Sexuality: A Nursing Perspective. Mcgraw-Hill Inc. New York, New York, 1980.

1.   Mims, 1980
2.   Comfort, 1972.

Happy Endings

The story of my relationship with the prostitute eventually had some happy endings. For one thing, I never again met a woman as bad as her. For another thing, I ended up getting a good job and earning back the money I lost and then some. Also, I met a black girl from a dating agency, and we quickly became friends. I took her to restaurants, the CN Tower, the art gallery, and we had a pretty good time. I was frustrated because she did not want to have sex, which I felt was probably because she did not like my lack of experience. Once, I tried to kiss her on the lips and she pushed me away, saying that she hated to kiss. I was very disappointed, but I later found out that it had nothing to do with her not liking me or even that she did not want to have sex with me. It was probably something that she learned from her culture.

One night, she asked if she could come over and go to a movie with me. I told her that I had no money at all because it was before payday, but I would be glad to cook for her. She said that she would be over in an hour and said good-bye.

I waited for her at the subway station, and when I saw her, I went up to her and we hugged. We went to my apartment, and I cooked orange chicken and Caribbean rice and beans for her. She said that it was good and that she wanted to look at my scholarship. I took her into the bedroom, and she looked at my scholarship and diplomas and clothes and went to sit on the bed. She surprised me with her next question.

"Want to see my breast?" she half asked, half stated.

"Yes," I blurted out, stunned.

Without further ado, she reached inside her dress and pulled out a beautiful big brown breast and held it up for me to look at for long moments. I knelt down and stared at this huge luscious breast, breathing heavily and unable to control my feelings. I'd never known her to be so brazen and sexy. Her breast was large, and full.

We walked to the subway hand in hand, and I put my arm around her, waiting for the bus. She got on it, and I called her to make sure she got home all right.

This was one of the most exciting moments of my limited sex life, and every time I thought about it, I got an erection.

We had several good experiences after that but eventually wound up parting—largely due to cultural differences and perhaps foolishness on the part of both of us. However, we always stayed good friends. I wound up helping her get a diploma in law and security administration, with a great deal of work on the part of both of us. The story gets better still.

Desiree

Desiree is one of the happiest endings to some of the sadder aspects of my life. I had so little confidence in myself as a man that I thought that I was either a homosexual or would become one. I later learned from the chief of sexology at the Clarke Institute that it is impossible to change your sexual preference. In order to be a homosexual, you must start out that way, and I knew that I had never been attracted to men until I was twenty-eight and that I was always strongly attracted to women. Dr. Kurt Freund of the Clarke Institute pointed out that human sexual nature is a bisexual nature. A heterosexual has a strong attraction to the opposite sex and a mild attraction to the same sex. Most people do not notice the mild attraction to the same sex because they do not focus on it. Noticing this mild attraction to the same sex can cause someone to worry and doubt himself. Incidentally, homosexuals have a mild attraction to the opposite sex, and some of them focus on it strongly and have sex with women so they say that they are bisexual. However, a true bisexual is someone who is almost equally attracted to both sexes. This is very rare. The number of people who are homosexual and call themselves bisexual is not as rare. Dr. Freund states that people do not choose their sexual preference, so we should not look down on someone who is different. The term "sexual preference" describes, well, human sexuality. We are not totally attracted to one sex and not at all attracted to the other, but rather have a strong preference for one sex over the other.

When I met Desiree, I fell in love and started to have regular intercourse with her and enjoyed it immensely. I knew that I was not a homosexual. Dr. Freund said that homosexuals can have sex with females, but for some reason, it does not register as pleasure. Desiree gave me much that is good in life. We shared love, sex, and many pleasures. We also shared both our joys and our sufferings.

At any rate, before I begin to talk about Desiree, let me say that if you think you might be a homosexual, you probably are not. If you really are a homosexual, try to adjust to it until a cure is found. Also, everyone should practice safe sex. Wear condoms, and do not have sex with anyone unless you are sure that they are HIV negative. Desiree and I both had the ELISA blood test for AIDS and are HIV negative.

One night, Desiree and I came home from one of the best movies I had ever seen, called *The Gods Must Be Crazy*. It was about bushmen who viewed men flying overhead as gods and found their behaviour to be somewhat strange. At 11:30 PM, we began to undress. She unbuttoned her blouse slowly. As I saw the cleft of her huge bosom, I walked over and touched it.

"That feels good," she said.

"It feels good to me too," I said.

She removed her blouse, then her skirt and panties, and finally her bra, fully revealing her 38DD breasts. She looked gorgeous. I looked at her and was glad that we had the foresight to buy condoms the day before. We had met her parents that day in a restaurant after going into the drug store because there was a sale on condoms. Her parents were very religious and strongly opposed to sex before marriage. We hid the condoms, and when they asked what we were doing in that area, rather than say that there was a sale on condoms, Desiree answered, "We wanted to see a special restaurant here."

At any rate, that night, Desiree lay naked on the bed with the sheet pulled up halfheartedly between her magnificent breasts, revealing more than it covered. The wiggle of her breasts when she moved and her all-round beauty gave me a throbbing erection. I quickly undressed and dressed up my organ in two condoms, one over the other. I took out some spermicidal cream and put it to one side. I knelt beside her while she lay naked on the bed and kissed her full on the lips while I felt her breast. It was so large that I could not get my hand close to covering all of it. I gave her a full body massage for a few minutes that eventually elicited a low moan of pleasure. I began to suck on her breasts, which got me even more excited. I then got on top of her and rubbed my penis between her breasts, making her nipples even more purple and swollen. I took out the spermicidal cream and applied it to her whole vagina and clitoris. I then began to massage her clitoris up and down in figure eights and a few other ways.

"I'm wet," she said. "Hurry up, Pete, I'm dying for it. Let's make love."

I climbed on top of her and rubbed my erect penis over her clitoris, causing her to again moan with pleasure. My penis then slid easily into her vagina. I began to thrust up and down, interspersed with kissing her lips and sucking on her breasts. After about thirty minutes of this, she reached her hand out to push me away, as if she'd had enough. We cuddled for five minutes.

After the five minutes, she said, "I want more."

I got on top of her and kissed her lips and felt her breast, giving me another erection. I slid into her vagina and went in and out of her for another half hour. I rubbed her breasts with my hairy chest, sucked on her breasts, and kissed her lips several times. Finally, she pushed me away, rolled on top of me and put her huge breasts over my penis, massaging my penis with her breasts. She then massaged my penis with her hand. We exchanged positions and made love until five thirty in the morning. Then we fell asleep in each other's arms and slept soundly for a few hours. I then went to the foam beside her bed and slept a little while longer. She woke me up to cuddle me with her soft body as we kissed and hugged and moved about together.

"I'm content," she said.

"Me too," I said.

She then made breakfast and said,

"Now our satisfaction is complete."

I found Desiree to be warm, loving, and affectionate and was glad that she persisted in chasing after me. At first, I thought that she was wrong for me because she had a developmental handicap and was legally blind. Later, I found out that she had a tremendous amount to offer. I take much pleasure in the way Desiree can rise to the occasion and lay aside her handicap. When we go to the Science Centre of Ontario, I enjoy showing her all the exhibits and explaining them, especially the biology exhibit. She takes it all in with great interest despite her handicaps. Desiree is a brave and delightful woman. I was very fortunate to have met Desiree and learned a good lesson about handicaps. Other people had used Desiree for sex or money or other things, and this was the first serious relationship for both of us. We shared so many experiences, sexual and otherwise that I can't even write them all down. After thirteen years, we continue to be very much in love. I think that the secret for both of us to finding and keeping a mate is to love someone by focusing on their good qualities. This will cause the person to love you back. It may not work every time, but it will work more often than not.

Dr. Cohen won a scholarship for having one of the
five highest marks in the university.
He has run thirty-three miles in six hours, swam five miles in three hours.
If he can change and you can change, then anybody can change.

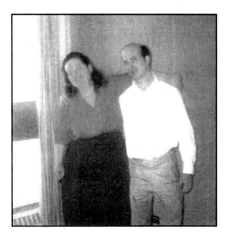

Diane and Dr. Pete at thirty.
(Mr. Pete) became Dr. Pete August 5, 1999 (age forty-six)

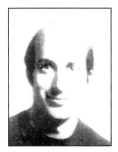

Pete at twenty-three.

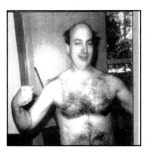

Dr. Pete at fifty.

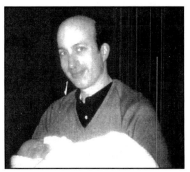

Dr. Pete at forty (Mr. Pete)

HOPE and HELP

for

KIDNEY FAILURE

by PETER COHEN, PhD

Candidate: Peter Cohen

Dissertation: Hope and Help for Kidney Failure

Quality of Scholarship:

This is an excellent piece of doctoral-level research and writing, one of
the better health care dissertations that I have read. It is evident that Mr.
Cohen has thoroughly researched this topic and integrated his findings
into the paper. Particularly interesting is the historical account of dialysis
as well as the discussion of bioartificial kidneys. This project is important
reading for any health care professional who deals with patients in renal
failure. The "pamphlet" section intended for patient reading is excellent
and should be produced in a professional manner with suitable graphics
and then made available to this patient population.

Adequacy of the Bibliography, Notes, Citations:

The bibliography is thorough, and key outcomes from the research are
utilized in the text. Mr. Cohen utilizes core textbooks in the field and
also incorporates current articles from the professional literature.

Writing, Language Use:

This is a very well-written and accurate discussion. I like the student's
direct literary style and feel that it is appropriate for a paper of this sort. I
would recommend that the document be published either as a reference
book or as a journal article in summary form.

Contents

Hope and Help for Kidney Failure–Abstract 65

Introduction 67

Review of the Literature 71

Procedures 89

Results and Summary 91

Appendix: Hope and Help for Kidney Failure 95

Kidney Failure and Its Treatment 97

Causes of Chronic Renal Failure 104

Other Treatments for Kidney Failure and Coping
with Kidney Failure 114

Future of Kidney-Failure Research 132

Bibliography 145

List of Illustrations

Normal Kidney 140

Nephron 141

Haemodialyser 142

Kidney Transplant 143

Bioartificial Kidney 144

Hope and Help for Kidney Failure– Abstract

This project is intended to give hope for the future to dialysis and kidney-failure patients and to help them cope with their problems before better treatments are available. It is a project in lieu of thesis and has six chapters plus an appendix. The first chapter is an introduction that tells why the project is so important, giving some statistics and stating the three main goals of the project. These are: helping a patient understand what is happening to his body, helping a patient cope with kidney failure, and finally to give hope for the future of kidney research. Chapters 2 and 3 are a review of the literature. The whole project is drawn heavily from the literature, and its originality comes from observing kidney failure firsthand and the fact that the whole is greater than the sum of its parts. I have never read a similar book. Chapter 4 deals with procedures, what was done to address the problem—mainly reviewing the literature in a unique way. Chapter 5 deals with results, findings, and summary, namely that kidney failure is difficult to cope with but can be helped with a positive attitude and good care. Chapter 6 deals with conclusions and recommendations. This chapter deals with how to increase hope for kidney patients, how fortunate people who have functioning kidneys are, and some suggestions for the future.

The appendix, is a short booklet for lay people to help patients and their families cope with kidney failure. Chapter 1 deals with normal anatomy, physiology, and pathology of the kidney. Chapter 2 deals with some treatments for kidney failure. Chapter 3 deals with hints for coping with kidney failure. Chapter 4 deals with psychological problems of kidney patients. Chapter 5 deals with the future of kidney failure research, drawing heavily from the work on the bioartificial kidney of Woods and Humes. It is intended to give kidney-failure patients something positive to think about.

Introduction

This project is on kidney failure and its treatment. The goal is to understand what is happening to the kidney-failure patient's body and the current treatments for it. Just as important, the second goal is to learn the best ways to cope with kidney failure and its psychological problems. Finally, the project will go into what will come next in the treatment of kidney failure, including some exciting research done by John Woods and David Humes on the making of a bioartificial kidney by tissue engineering. Being able to make an artificial kidney could solve the problem of the shortage of kidneys for transplants, as well as solving many other problems for people with kidney failure.

There is a great need for a work of this type. There are few, if any, books that deal with all aspects of hope and help for kidney failure. Some books deal with one aspect of kidney failure but do not cover a broad spectrum of problems. It is estimated that 250,000 people in the United States suffer from kidney failure, referred to as end-stage renal disease (ESRD). They depend on dialysis or a kidney transplant to stay alive (Schnermann, 1998, p.7). In Toronto, Canada, there is a five hundred-person waiting list for kidney transplants, and it can take five years or more to get a kidney transplant. About one hundred kidney transplants are done each year (Cole, 1998).

I have selected to undertake this problem because I am acutely aware of the problems facing kidney patients as I have a close friend with kidney failure. There has been much progress made with treating kidney failure, but it is still very difficult. Patients on long-term dialysis have an approximately 30% survival rate, and their mortality rate is similar to that of some cancers (Schnermann, 1998, p. 8). Hopefully, better treatments for kidney failure will be found.

As mentioned, there are very few books written for the layman on coping with and having hope for kidney failure, so this paper will be very welcome to patients and their families. Very often, loved ones are the silent, untreated victims of someone's illness. This paper will address that problem, from someone who has been in that situation.

The problem of kidney failure raises a number of questions in the patient's mind such as:

"Will I die?"

"What are my chances of leading a normal life?"

"This regimen is very rigorous. Can I stick to it?"

"What does the future hold for me?"

I have seen dialysis patients handle their worries and problems with great courage. There is a viewpoint held by some psychologists that living itself takes courage (Lacome, 1998). Kidney-failure patients especially need this courage and a will to live. Some people give up their dialysis routines and let themselves die. This paper is intended to minimize that occurrence and show dialysis patients that they are not alone, and that there is hope for a much brighter future. Dialysis is often painful because the person must be stuck with needles for four hours, three times per week. The dietary restrictions, such as few high-potassium foods, can be very distressing to some people. This can lead to more psychological problems. There is a certain knack to coping with kidney failure. This paper will try to address these issues.

Again, I must stress that the hope for better treatments is possible. I hope that the researchers, especially John Woods and David Humes, will be successful in developing a bioartificial kidney to give more quality and quantity of life to a kidney patient.

All hemodialysis patients need to have an artery joined to a vein or have a graft added to give access for putting the dialysis needles into the patient. If this process, which is called vascular access, develops a clot, as often happens, a very painful declotting procedure must be done, called balloon angioplasty. This involves puncturing the skin and artery with a sharp instrument and putting a catheter into the artery in order to press the clot into the vein, thus rendering it harmless. If a clot develops in vascular access, it cannot be used for dialysis and a catheter must be inserted into one of the large arteries of the legs, shoulders or breasts. If these arteries are used too frequently, they will not function and the patient may run out of options. This is another reason why kidney patients need better treatments. Kidney-failure patients and their families should try to find out about and support kidney research.

It will be shown in this paper how important the kidneys are in maintaining human life and contribute to many functions of the body. This is another reason why kidney failure is such an important topic. I once read an article in the *Toronto Star* about a young girl in kidney failure who fractured her arm just by moving it. This happened because the kidneys play a great role in calcium and phosphate metabolism, and patients can have very weakened bones.

This project must be considered as a whole. Sometimes questions will arise, or an explanation will seem incomplete because it is explained in more detail later in the project.

Review of the Literature

The review of the literature will be very extensive. Some parts will be repeated in a different form in the appendix. There are two parts to the review of the literature. One deals with what is going on presently, and the other deals with future research. There are two terms for kidneys. One is *nephro* from the Greek word *nephros*, meaning "kidney," and the other is *renal*, from the Latin word *renes*, meaning "kidneys" (Cameron, 1996, p.4).

The first useful dialysis machine was made by a Dutch physician named Willem Johan Kolff who asserted that even without hope, you should persevere. He was tenacious and had a quest to heal. Kolff learned some of these qualities from his father who confided that he felt helpless as he watched a patient dying (Douglis, 1988, p. 282).

When the younger Kolff was a twenty-seven-year-old physician working towards his PhD at the University of Groningen, he cared for his first patient dying of kidney failure. The young farmer had lost his sight and vomited repeatedly, as wastes normally excreted by the kidneys and eliminated in the urine accumulated in his blood. Kolff was heartbroken at having to tell the man's elderly mother that her son was about to die. Kolff thought, "If only I could remove twenty grams of the waste product, urea, from the patient's body each day, the man might live (Douglis, 1988, p. 282)."

Scientists before Kolff had tried unsuccessfully to build machines that would cleanse the blood. In 1938, a biochemistry professor introduced Kolff to the wonders of cellophane (Douglis, 1988, p. 282). Kolff filled a sausagelike cellophane casing with blood and urea and swished the tubing in saltwater. Within five minutes, all the urea had passed through the cellophane membrane into the water, while the blood remained in the casing. The blood had been purified or dialysed.

Kolff persevered while patient after patient died subsequent to using his primitive dialysis machines made of aluminum drums partially immersed in saltwater. He tinkered with the technique until, finally, in 1945, he saved the life of a sixty-seven-year-old woman: dialysis patient number 17.

Kolff was so eager to share his invention with the world that he shipped his machines, unpatented, to hospitals in London, New York, and Montreal. When he emigrated to the United States and joined the Cleveland Clinic in 1950, Kolff adapted a Maytag washing machine for home dialysis. He then went on to develop other artificial organs (Douglis, 1988, p. 282).

Some Considerations in Chronic Renal Failure

The prognosis for patients with kidney failure and diabetes is considerably worse than for patients with kidney failure who are not diabetic. This prognosis is particularly poor for elderly patients. Fewer than one in ten of the two thousand diabetics over sixty-five who began dialysis were alive after five years. These diabetics were usually sick, mostly with cardiovascular disease, before they developed ESRD. Also, patients with renal vascular disease fared almost as poorly (Locatelli, 1998, p. 381).

One important factor in ESRD patients is to maintain good control of blood sugar and hypertension. These two conditions damage the heart, blood vessels, and brain. Uremia itself also tends to damage the heart and blood vessels so that it is important to maintain general health and keep hemoglobin levels as high as possible (Locatelli, 1998, p. 382). Poor nutritional status is also a problem with diabetics (Locatelli, 1998 p. 381). By the time a diabetic patient undergoes dialysis, he has had a buildup of uremia toxins for several years together with anemia, metabolic acidosis, and hyperparathyroidism—all symptoms of kidney failure. It is best to have as little underlying disease process as possible when the patient begins renal replacement therapy (RRT) (Locatelli, 1998, p. 382). The earlier someone with kidney failure is referred to RRT, the better his prognosis.

It used to be that high-risk patients such as the elderly, diabetics, HIV-positive, and others were not referred to nephrologists when they went into kidney failure. Now, nephrologists give RRT to anyone who needs it (Locatelli, 1998, p. 383). The European doctors are still selective about who they refer for RRT. Javex, a disinfectant, effectively kills all infection, even viruses that might get into the dialysis machine so that patients are protected from contracting HIV or hepatitis B or C from dialysis (Erica Macdonald, a nurse on dialysis, 1998).

It is best to start dialysis early. Studies have shown that patients who start dialysis before they have a great deal of ESRD symptoms do better and live longer (Locatelli, 1998, p. 384). The criteria for starting RRT is high creatinine levels in the blood, elevated blood urea nitrogen (BUN), albumen in the urine and the inability to excrete creatinine.

Kidney transplantation is done on patients who have the best prognosis. It is not done on patients with a poor prognosis, who must remain on dialysis. Transplantation significantly increases the life expectancy and quality of life for ESRD patients and is the best therapy for many patients.

Old age gives the worst prognosis for ESRD patients. They are more likely to have other diseases, such as heart disease, cerebral vascular disease, and other co-morbid diseases. Hypertension is another risk factor that can shorten the life of an ESRD patient. It is a major cause of heart disease and makes attendance at dialysis imperative because dialysis draws off excess fluid that can raise the blood pressure and overstrain the heart (Locatelli, 1998, p. 387).

Anemia is a major cause of heart failure, also caused by kidney failure, and is treated with erythropoietin (EPO). EPO causes the bone marrow to create more red blood cells, and relieves some of the anemia (Locatelli, 1998, p. 388). However, a kidney-failure patient seldom has more than two-thirds of his hemoglobin restored.

Hemodialysis can cause a breakdown of body proteins. It is controversial whether the kidney-failure patient should get more or less protein since protein, in excess, is broken down to urea and places a strain on the liver and kidneys. The most recent belief is that more protein is better because some protein is lost in dialysis (Locatelli, 1998, p. 389).

If patients have been given anti-inflammatory steroids, such as prednisone, it greatly increases their susceptibility to infection as well as the risk of malignancies.

Heart disease and kidney disease go hand-in-hand. More than 50% of the deaths in kidney patients are due to cardiovascular disorders, which are present at the start of dialysis therapy.

Anemia is a risk factor for heart disease. It is common among kidney patients because they do not produce erythropoietin. Treating the anemia with EPO greatly decreases the incidence of cardiovascular disorders (Locatelli, 1998, p. 389).

Lack of calcium and excess of phosphates with secondary hyperparathyroidism (excess of activity in the parathyroid glands) are characteristics of ESRD. The parathyroid glands secrete parathyroid hormone, which is responsible for maintaining calcium balance in the body. Calcium levels affect almost all cell processes. It is excess phosphates that cause the development and progression of secondary hyperparathyroidism because they compete with calcium. This is another factor that contributes to morbidity and mortality among dialysis patients (Locatelli, 1998, p. 390).

Excess sodium removal and low blood pressure during dialysis may contribute to problems with dialysis patients. Also, trying to do dialysis too quickly with too great a flow rate is dangerous. These factors all contribute to the mortality of dialysis patients, particularly among the elderly (Locatelli, 1998, p. 390).

Increasing Life Span of Patients with Exercise

Exercise may be helpful in increasing the life span of dialysis patients and their quality of life (Mercer, 1998, p. 2023). Walking tests may be useful to assess the fitness of dialysis patients. They are easy to administer, are well tolerated by patients, and give meaningful results (Mercer, 1998, p. 2023). Stair climbing is also a good test of fitness for dialysis patients.

A study was done in which walking scores were correlated with stair climbing and cycle ergometer tests to measure fitness in dialysis patients. Peak oxygen uptake is the most frequently employed method of describing exercise intolerance in studies of patients with ESRD. Walking tests measure capability as well as peak oxygen uptake and are cheaper and easier to administer than conventional methods of testing peak oxygen uptake (Mercer, 1998, p. 2024). Walking and stair climbing tests correlated accurately with cycle ergometer and more traditional methods of measuring maximal oxygen uptake. The study was done on twenty-five healthy dialysis patients, eighteen hemodialysis patients, and seven peritoneal dialysis patients. Walking and stair-climbing tests were administered after previously having done the more traditional cycle ergometer tests for maximal oxygen uptake (Mercer, 1998, 2024).

The walking and stair-climbing test measured the time in seconds to walk fifty meters in length and twenty-two 0.015-meter steps. Time was measured with a stopwatch, and the BORG method of perceived exertion was used in addition to other methods. The BORG method of perceived exertion measures how hard the subject feels he is working on a scale of 1 to 20. The standard error of the estimate was 11% (Mercer, 1998, p. 2024).

The results were that peak oxygen uptake correlated strongly between the walk and stair-climb test and the traditional cycle ergometer test (Mercer, 1998, p. 2025). Therefore, it is best and safest to use a walk and stair-climb test to measure fitness in ESRD patients. People should not take the test if they have heart disease, unless it has been approved by their physician. See appendix for more information.

Kidney Transplants

Kidney transplants are still the best treatment for ESRD. The main problem with transplantation is rejection and antirejection drugs that must be administered in order to counteract this. Antirejection treatment with monoclonal antibodies has been undertaken, mostly with poor success. This poor success has been mostly due to the terrible side effects of monoclonal antibodies. For example, the monoclonal antibody, OKT3 causes fever, chills, tremor, shortness of breath, chest pains, nausea, vomiting, diarrhea, headache, muscle and bone pain, brain inflammation (meningitis), and, most serious of all, pulmonary edema (fluid in the lungs). Pulmonary edema can be treated by dialysis or diuretics and the other symptoms can be treated by administering prednisolone six hours before the OKT3 (monoclonal antibody) therapy, and another dose one hour before the OKT3 therapy. Diuretics do not work well among kidney patients because they have little or no kidney function.

If the treatment with monoclonal antibodies can be refined and perfected, it may be very helpful in preventing rejection of a transplanted organ. Monoclonal antibodies are not so useful now. They work by increasing levels of interleukin-2 and other cytokines in the body, but are highly toxic (Schena, 1997, pp. 55-58).

Progression of Kidney Failure in Diabetic Nephropathy

The factors that are involved in progression from diabetes mellitus to kidney failure, called diabetic nephropathy, are important to know. They are: genetic predisposition, hereditary factors, and the early appearance of microalbumenuria (albumen in the urine that can only be detected by a microscope). Systemic high blood pressure, high blood sugar, and smoking also play a role in kidney failure, according to Carmelita Maccantoni (Maccontoni, 1998, p. 16). It appears that the main mechanisms behind diabetic nephropathy destroying the kidneys are:

(1) Activation of protein kinase C.
(2) Non-enzymatic glycation of various matrix proteins and their accumulation in the kidneys.
(3) Stimulation of several growth factors, overstimulating and damaging kidney function.
(4) Generation of reactive oxygen substances.
(5) Stimulation of collagen biosynthesis (Maccontoni, 1998, p. 18).

Systemic Hypertension

High blood pressure is a well-known cause of kidney failure and damage to the kidneys. When the mean arterial pressure (MAP) is too high, it scars and damages kidney tissue. That is why everyone, especially diabetics, should have their blood pressure kept within normal limits, with medication if necessary (Maccontoni, 1998, p. 16).

With NIDDM, high blood pressure is a frequent finding, and it may precede or follow diabetic nephropathy. With this diabetic kidney disease, or diabetic nephropathy, many additional factors including blood vessel disease complications, insulin resistance, and intolerance of body lipids (fats) can cause kidney damage. Insulin resistance is most often caused by obesity. Obesity is defined as having more than 30% excess body fat. The insulin secreted by the pancreas has too much area to service and so it cannot work properly (Maccontoni, 1998, p. 16).

It has also been found in studies among Pima Indians that the higher the blood pressure, the greater the chance of having albumen in the urine when diabetes struck (Maccontoni, 1998 p. 16). Diastolic blood pressure was the most important factor in whether or not kidney damage was done, but MAP, mean arterial pressure was important too. Diastolic blood pressure is the pressure in the arteries when the heart is relaxed and so is lower because the heart is not forcing blood through the arteries. Systolic blood pressure is the pressure when the heart is contracted and is the high figure because the heart is forcefully pumping blood through the arteries. Mean arterial pressure is the average between the two. People with the highest blood pressure showed the greatest decline in glomerular filtration rate, GFR, when they developed diabetes (ibid, p. 16). GFR is the amount of blood processed by the filtering, blood vessel-like part of the kidney, the glomerulus.

Predictors of Kidney Failure

Microalbumenuria is the presence of albumen in the urine that can only be detected by a microscope. It is an ominous sign and is an indication that kidney failure is coming. Several therapeutic measures, such as dietary protein restriction, sugar control, and medication to treat high blood pressure can often partially reverse diabetic nephropathy for a while. Protein restriction is controversial. These measures, also, may only postpone the inevitable (Maccontoni, 1998, p. 17). Microalbumenuria is also a risk factor for heart disease. Protein in the urine is the worst sign that chronic renal failure is near (Maccontoni, 1998 p. 17).

High blood sugar is another cause of kidney failure because glycose-protein end products get deposited in the micro-circulation of the kidneys and damage them (Maccontoni, 1998, p. 17).

Excess growth factor excess is a cause of kidney failure. This can be explained by the fact that growth factors can damage the kidneys by causing their cells to swell. Again, diabetes mellitus is the cause of excess growth factor secretion (Maccontoni, 1998 p. 17). The process of glycosylated protein end products being created is a complex chemical reaction that is difficult to explain to a non-chemist and is called the Maillard reaction (Maccontoni, 1998, p. 17).

Excess angiotensin 2 has also been shown to damage the kidneys by causing swelling of kidney tissue (ibid, p. 18). Hyperglycaemia will aggravate kidney damage along with this effect. Once kidney failure sets in, it progresses more rapidly because of the swelling caused by the renin-angiotensin2 factors.

The Importance of Decreasing Diabetic Nephropathy in NIDDM Patients

Diabetic nephropathy has become the leading cause of ESRD in many countries in Western Europe, similar to the USA. It used to be thought that the risk of developing kidney failure with NIDDM was small. Now, findings are that NIDDM is the greatest cause of kidney failure. It has now turned out that 40% of people receiving renal replacement therapy had their kidney failure caused by NIDDM. My friend lost her kidney function three years after developing type 2 diabetes mellitus (NIDDM).

Part of the reason for more NIDDM patients going into kidney failure is because society as a whole is aging and older people are more likely to go into kidney failure, according to Ritz (1998, p. 6). Ritz also says that people with type 2 diabetes mellitus are living longer due to improved medical care. I find these explanations difficult to believe because my friend was only forty-five when she developed kidney failure.

The problem of ESRD in patients with NIDDM can be prevented somewhat by anti-hypertensive treatment, particularly with angiotensin constrictive enzyme (ACE) blockers, intensified control of blood sugar, cessation of smoking, lipid (fat) lowering and possibly lowering of protein intake. Protein, in excess has to be broken down to urea by the liver and then excreted by the kidneys. This can overload the kidneys (Ritz, 1998, pp. 6-10). My friend had all these beneficial effects of medical care, but went into kidney failure in spite of her good medical care. Her original kidney doctor said that she would have no problem if she lost sixty pounds, which would reverse her diabetes. This upset her so much that she went on an eating binge and she actually put on weight. Obesity is a major cause of NIDDM.

Anatomy and Physiology of the Kidney

The kidney has many functions necessary to the body. See appendix for more details. The functions that are unique to the kidney itself are two-fold. One is filtration and excretion and the other is reabsorption. Filtration is accomplished by the glomerulus of the nephron. The nephron is a tiny functional unit of the kidney, each of which has 1.2 million. This shows how tiny a nephron is because a kidney is only the size of someone's fist. The tubules, consisting of the proximal convoluted tubule, the loop of Henle and the distal convoluted tubules are responsible for reabsorbing necessary substances. They also are placed along the nephron in the order given. The dialysis machine only accomplishes the filtration function of the kidney. The reabsorbing function of the kidney is duplicated only in the plans for Woods and Humes's bioartificial kidney. Both the filtration and reabsorbing parts are tubular in shape and do not look like a kidney at all. The bioartificial kidney has worked in small animals, but must be refined before it is ready for implanting into humans, estimated at two and a half years from now (Cutler, 1998,).

Kidney Diseases

Kidney failure can be caused by a variety of diseases. The most common cause is diabetes mellitus. Other causes are hypertension and autoimmune diseases, such as systemic lupus erythematosis, a disease in which the body attacks its own immune system. Among the diseases that can cause kidney failure are:

(A) *Prerenal Diseases*—These are diseases in which other systemic diseases affect the kidneys. Among them are:
  (1) Volume depletion. This includes dehydration and shock in which the kidney does not get enough blood and so malfunctions.
  (2) Heart failure.
  (3) Liver cirrhosis.
  (4) Nephrotic syndrome, structural disorders of the renal arteries, and blood vessels.
  (5) Low blood pressure, so that the kidneys do not get enough blood.
  (6) Renal artery narrowing.

(B) *Intrarenal Diseases*—These are diseases inside the kidneys. Some of them can be reversed if treated early enough. The main group of intrarenal diseases are vascular diseases. Among them are vasculitis, an inflammation of the blood vessels in the kidneys. Hypertension in the kidneys is another cause of kidney failure. Scarring of the kidneys and clots in the kidneys can also cause kidney failure. Glomerulonephritis, an inflammation of the kidneys can cause kidney failure. Dying of the tubules, cancer, too much blood calcium, too much uric acid, cysts on the kidneys, giving the wrong medications and aspirin and other nonsteroidal anti-inflammatory drugs can cause kidney failure.

(C) *Post-Renal Disease*—is a disease of the organs that the kidneys drain into. Among them are:
  (1) Obstructive uropathy, usually obstruction of the ureters going into the bladder.
  (2) Prostatic disease, such as prostate cancer.
  (3) Kidney stones.

There are about eighty different kidney diseases that can cause kidney failure. Some of these do not cause kidney failure if treated properly and promptly, including glomerulonephritis, pyelonephritis, hypercalcemia, and uric acid nephropathy. Uric acid nephropathy is an excess of uric acid in the blood, which is damaging the kidneys. Uric acid is an end-product of cell reproduction and can be gotten rid of with allopurinol, a drug made from an enzyme in the body that breaks down uric acid (McPhee, 1997, pp. 386-391).

Signs of Kidney Failure

One of the early signs of kidney failure is what used to be called dropsy. It is a swelling of any part of the body that is left dependent—that is, lower in position than the heart (Cameron, 1996, p. 19). This ailment is now called edema and is a sign that the body is not getting rid of fluid properly. Pain is not a frequent sign of kidney failure because internal organs such as kidneys do not feel pain (Cameron, 1996, p. 20).

Other signs of kidney failure are tiredness due to low hemoglobin, pallor from the same dry itchy skin due to poisons not being excreted by the kidneys, and bone problems because no calcitriol is being secreted by the kidneys (Cameron, 1996, p. 21). Calcitriol is the hormone that raises blood calcium.

Tests for albumen and protein in the urine are helpful for determining impending kidney failure, especially when done on a twenty-four-hour urine collection. When a patient goes into frank and complete kidney failure, urine tests are not helpful because the person excretes little or no urine. After that, blood tests for urea, creatinine, potassium, hemoglobin, phosphates, and calcium become essential. Rising creatinine and urea in the blood are signs of kidney failure (Cameron, 1996 p. 23).

In Britain, about seven thousand people each year reach ESRD. Forty to fifty thousand people in Britain have kidney failure or a disease that will cause it. About half of these people will be over seventy (Cameron, 1996, p. 29). The drug phenacetin has been found to damage the kidneys in most people, and most countries have banned this drug (Cameron, 1996, p. 50). Also, drugs such as aspirin reduce circulation to the kidneys, putting a strain on kidney function.

It was mentioned that systemic lupus erythematosus can cause kidney failure, and this is a simple case of the body attacking its own kidney (Cameron, 1996, p. 51). This disease can either burn out or require dialysis.

Amyloidosis is a common cause of kidney failure as well. Amyloid is an insoluble group of proteins that can damage body organs, especially the kidneys. These can be triggered by infections or inflammations such as those that occur with rheumatoid arthritis or bone infection (osteomyelitis). Amyloidosis seldom appears before age fifty (Cameron, 1996, p.65).

It is important for a kidney patient not to take in too much phosphate because the parathyroids secrete more parathyroid hormone to counter excess phosphate. The result is bone disease, and the patient can become overrun by calcium phosphate, also called chalk (Cameron, 1996, p. 73). Calcium and phosphate are mutually antagonistic, and bone problems can occur if too much phosphorus is consumed. Calcium carbonate (chalk) helps raise lowered calcium and binds phosphate (Cameron, 1996, p. 80).

Cameron asserts that since 1996, it has been well established that a low-protein diet has very little effect in ameliorating kidney disease (Cameron, 1996, p. 79) as has been suggested by many people, some of whom were quoted in this project.

What Dialysis Entails

With dialysis, first, blood is taken out of the body from blood vessels and is treated with an anticoagulant to prevent it from clotting when in contact with the plastics and surfaces outside the body. The blood is then pumped into a dialyser where it passes over semipermeable membranes (usually made of cellulose), and an exchange of dissolved substances takes place. The exchange occurs across the membrane and from a solution called dialysate, whose composition is determined by those doing dialysis and according to patient need. The makeup of this fluid approximates to an ideal solution of the body's salts dissolved in water. It need not be sterile because the dialysis membrane is too thick to allow bacteria through, although some products from dead bacteria can penetrate and cause problems on occasion. The dialysis solution takes out harmful substances and then circulates the blood back into the blood vessels (Cameron, 1996, pp.85-87). Water is removed by suction, called ultrafiltration (Cameron, 1996, p. 88). Water and its dissolved salts are passed through the membrane. The pressure on the other side is lowered by a pump, which suctions off water (Cameron, 1996, p. 88).

An arteriovenous fistula, in which an artery is joined to a vein and becomes toughened by having the needle put in is used to draw off and return blood for haemodialysis. This is called vascular access (Cameron, 1996, p. 90).

Typical Medications for Dialysis Patients

(1) Iron to combat anaemia.
(2) Vitamins because some are lost in the dialyser.
(3) Phosphate-binders such as calcium carbonate, since protein foods contain phosphate, and too much blood phosphate makes acid blood. Calcium carbonate, when taken on an empty stomach increases blood calcium. When it is taken with food, just after eating, it binds phosphate, in addition to raising blood calcium.
(4) Calcitriol to aid in maintaining strong bones with a more normal calcium metabolism.
(5) Blood pressure medication if necessary.
(6) EPO to maintain red blood cell count and combat anaemia.
(7) Laxatives if necessary.
(8) Diabetic medications or insulin to maintain acceptable blood sugar levels for diabetics (Cameron, 1996, p. 100).

Diet

While on hemodialysis, you must restrict your fluid intake to two and one half cups or 500 ml. This is drawn off by hemodialysis at each session (Cameron, 1996, p. 101).

It is important to take in enough protein to make muscle and other tissue because some protein is lost during dialysis. However, many proteins contain phosphates, so it is important to take phosphate binders, such as calcium carbonate (Cameron, 1996, p. 101).

Salt intake needs to be watched because this can lead to fluid retention and high blood pressure. Potassium also needs to be restricted. However, even with all these restrictions, there are many tasty foods that can be eaten (Cameron, 1996, p. 102).

Some Psychological Problems of Dialysis Patients

There are many psychological problems faced by dialysis patients. See appendix for more details. Cameron calls psychological problems, "the most important problems of all faced by patients on long-term dialysis (Cameron, 1996, p. 104)."

The most serious problem is expressed or unexpressed suicide. Different persons come to terms with long-term dialysis in different ways. Individual temperaments, degree of family support, or job are all factors in adjustment to dialysis and kidney-failure regimens. Patients who accept situations without complaint have a great deal of family support and have meaningful work that they can do, fare better than people who do not have these supports. My friend has good support from her mother and her sisters, a job that she can work at whenever she wants to, and an acceptance of her fate. She sometimes becomes depressed, as she admits, but has never been suicidal and soon gets over feeling depressed when something good happens.

Some marriages break up because of a family member on dialysis, and the stress of kidney failure is usually felt by all members of the family. Other families do not break up because of dialysis but are more securely welded because of it (Cameron, 1996, p. 105).

Depression, sexual impotence in men, and lack of sexual urge in females are common complaints. Tiredness due to anemia as well as the hormonal changes of kidney failure aggravate these problems. Earnings frequently go down, jobs become harder to get, money worries pile up, and social life might be limited due to tiredness (Cameron, 1996, p. 105).

Having to dialyse three times a week is a severe source of stress. The patient may have fears of something going wrong with dialysis, fears of death, and fear of a layman botching dialysis if it is done at home. Aggressive behavior and noncompliance with food and fluid restrictions are signs of psychological problems. Cameron advocates mutual patient support groups in order to help people with psychological problems (1996, p. 105).

History of Kidney Transplantation

Transplanting organs became theoretically possible in the early 1900s when doctors learned to remove organs from one person and transfer them to another. However, the most that these transplants lasted was a few months and then the organs were destroyed and the patient died. Eventually, they found that transplants with identical twins were successful and lasted for thirty years or more. The doctors soon learned that rejection of the transplanted organ was the problem. The immune system recognized the transplanted organ as something foreign and attacked it. The transplants with identical twins began in the 1950s.

In 1962, the new drug azathiopurine (Imuran) was shown to be very effective in combating rejection, especially when given in conjunction with prednisone. The doctor mainly had to respect the ABO, Rh blood-typing system. People with Rh negative blood can only receive kidneys from other people with Rh negative blood. People with Rh positive blood can receive kidneys from Rh negative and positives. Type A blood can receive blood and kidneys from A and O. Type B can receive blood from B and O. Type AB can receive blood from A,B,AB, and O, and type O can receive blood only from O.

By 1965, transplants with people who had just died were successful. Cyclosporine brought a higher success rate among transplant patients so that 84% of transplants were successful after the first year and 75% of transplants still worked after five years. There is still room for improvement and John Woods and David Humes's bioartificial kidney might be the answer (Cameron, 1996, pp. 122-123).

The Future of Kidney Research

This project's goal is to help people understand kidney failure and its treatment better, and to help people cope with kidney failure. Finally, hope for the future is the third goal of the project.

Xenotransplantation, which is a transplant from another species to a human, has previously resulted in failure and destruction of the foreign organ in ten days. It started to become successful when researchers were able to transplant a human gene into a pig's ovary, then take a kidney or a liver and transplant it into a human (Abraham, 1999). If the human gene was taken from the person needing the transplant, the xenotransplantation might be even more successful.

A South Korean team tried the same experiment as tried above, but after implanting human DNA into an animal with both a human egg and sperm, they stopped because of ethical concerns. This approach has shown promise (*Toronto Star*, 1998).

Scientific American describes the same process of implanting a human gene into an animal embryo (Wilmot, 1999, pp. 58-63). Pulses of electric current were given to a human egg after it was put on a Petri dish. The electrical impulses caused growth, simulating a sperm. They then implanted this cloned group of cells into a sheep. These experiments can make human stem cells and these can be transplanted into humans and conceivably grow into a viable organ. This research came from making Dolly, the cloned sheep. It may solve the problem of lack of human donors (Wilmot, 1998, pp.58-63).

Stem cells are undifferentiated cells that grow and replace damaged organ cells. This is another answer to the problem of kidney failure (Fox, 1998, p. 76). Stem cells are taken from human fetuses without harming them, however, the technique has not been perfected (Fox, 1998, p. 76).

Discover science magazine reports that two laboratories working on privately funded research, reported that they isolated human embryonic stem cells, which can give rise to many organs in the body. The hope is to grow customised tissue to replace cells and organs lost to disease, including the kidneys (Morell, 1998, p.84)

In the early stages of embryonic development, cells are undifferentiated, and over the course of time, develop into specialised cells that perform specific functions. When scientists captured undifferentiated human embryonic cells, called stem cells, with embryos donated for research by couples undergoing in vitro fertilisation, they knew they had the start of a tool to make new organs. The one problem with this approach is that scientists do not yet know how to make a stem cell grow into the organ that they want. This article shows that progress is being made into that area (Richardson, 1999, pp. 58-60).

In an earlier issue of *Discover* magazine, Joseph Vacanti, a researcher at Children's Hospital in Boston, created a liver by using wads of spongelike biodegradable polymers. Vacanti has managed to make a circulatory system for his tiny artificial livers. Blood vessel cells and liver cells manage to sort themselves out and go to the right places.

This process could conceivably be done with kidneys in order to create a laboratory-grown kidney. This would be a form of tissue engineering similar to what John Woods and David Humes are doing. However, the work of Woods and Humes is much more promising. It will be discussed in detail in the appendix. Woods and Humes have been working on the problem of a tissue-engineered kidney for many years (Pool, May, 1998, p.52).

Reasons for Kidney Patients to be Hopeful

Tissue engineering is a rapidly growing field in biotechnology. The use and packaging of synthetic materials, biologic compounds, and cellular components of specific tissues can replace the function of diseased organs. The kidney was the first organ to have its function replaced by a machine (dialysis). The kidney was the first organ to be transplanted, and the kidney may be the first organ in which tissue engineering concepts will produce an implantable device for replacement of that organ's functions. In order to replace blood ultrafiltration performed by renal glomeruli and reabsorption performed by renal tubules, a tubular-looking device was considered six years ago. This device, when perfected, would increase life expectancy, increase the patient's ability to move about, increase quality of life, and save the patient's time so that he need not go for dialysis, lessen the risk of infection, and reduce costs. This approach would be considered a cure rather than a treatment (Humes, 1993, p.678). This bioartificial kidney has already been implanted into small animals (1998) and just needs to be scaled up in order to be implanted into humans. Humes estimates that this will be done in two years, and five years later, the device can be mass-produced after extensive testing (Humes, 1998).

In 1993, it was found that it was possible to grow kidney stem cells from the proximal tubules of adult mammalian kidneys. This is why kidneys can recover from severe injury. The trick in 1993 was to harness that quality. Now, there is every indication that tubular cells can grow into any part of the tubules, such as the proximal tubule, the loop of Henle, or the distal tubule. The section on anatomy and physiology of the kidney explains what these parts do and will be discussed further in the appendix. Blood vessel cells can be used to make a glomerulus for filtration.

Using renal proximal tubule cells in primary culture, it has been found that the growth factors TGF-B and EGF, along with the retinoid, retinoic acid, promoted growth of tubule progenitor cells in tissue culture. This is considered a major indication that it is possible to duplicate renal tubular function. The methodology to purify and grow renal tubular progenitor cells allows for the possibility to provide better therapeutic alternatives to current expensive medical substitution therapies for the treatment of ESRD by replacing filtering, regulatory and endocrine functions of kidney tissue (Humes, 1993, p.679).

It is important to note that replacement of kidney functions means replacement of the filtering unit, the glomerulus, and the regulatory unit, the tubule. Together, they form the basic component of the kidney, called the nephron. A bioartificial kidney requires two main components: glomeruli and renal tubules.

Bioartificial Glomerulus

The potential for a bioartificial glomerulus has been achieved with the use of polysulphone fibers outside the body that lasts for six weeks. The availability of hollow fibers with high permeability has been an important advancement in biomaterials for replacement function of glomerular ultrafiltration (Humes, 1993, p. 679). There is a maintenance of pressure in this bioartificial glomerulus for the purpose of moving fluid in and out for ultrafiltration. Most of the problems for building an artificial glomerulus can be overcome (Humes, 1993, p. 679).

Another reason why a bioartificial glomerulus can be created is the fact that extracellular matrix, a part of kidneys, can be produced by MDCK cells and can produce the holes necessary to move fluids in and out of the bioartificial kidney.

Bioartificial Tubule

"The bioartificial renal tubule is clearly feasible when conceived as a combination of living cells supported on polymeric substrata." (Humes, 1993, p. 680). This is the whole idea of tissue engineering. It means creating a structure with a combination of an artificial infrastructure and living cells on its support. A bioartificial proximal tubule may work so well in providing all the functions of the kidney such as reabsorption, hormone secretion, and regulation of fluid balance that other parts of the kidney like the loop of Henle will not be necessary (Humes, 1993, p. 686).

An Implantable Artificial Kidney

An implantable bioartificial kidney is feasible because the filtration device (glomerulus) and the tubule unit are feasible. There will be no problem of rejection because the foreign cells will be encapsulated with synthetic polymers and therefore inaccessible to attack by the host's immune system (which means that antirejection drugs will not be necessary. This is an important goal of the implantable bioartificial kidney (ibid, p. 680).

The bioartificial kidney would most likely be hooked up to the patient's iliac arteries and veins and would be in tubular, rather than kidney-shaped form. It would be done similarly to a kidney transplant, with all the advantages mentioned above.

Stewart Cameron says that the possibility of growing whole kidneys in the laboratory from human cells, perhaps even from the cells of the person needing the treatment "is attractive but immensely complicated." He says that the problem is that we do not know the structure of the template that the DNA carries which tells the mass of cells which are to become a kidney to organise themselves into one. He says, "However, in theory it should be possible." (Cameron, 1996, p. 203). Apparently, he is not familiar with the North American work on tissue engineering. It is not necessary to know exact DNA replicas of kidneys, although with the human genome project that maps out human genes, to be completed in the year 2003 even that might be possible. I was very encouraged by the work of Woods, Humes, and Cieslinski.

I believe that in this review of the literature, I have answered the three main objectives of my project. One is to help people know more kidney failure and what is happening to their bodies, which will be dealt with in greater detail in the appendix. The second goal is to show people that they can cope with kidney failure, knowing the psychological problems that it can cause. It will also be dealt with in greater detail in the appendix. The third goal was to show the immense hope that kidney research holds for people with kidney failure.

Procedures

This chapter will describe what I have done to address the problem of kidney failure. It is only fitting to describe the problem first. My first problem was to explain the normal function and structure of the kidney in order to explain to kidney-failure patients what is happening to their bodies. I also dealt with some of the diseases that can cause kidney failure and the medical considerations of kidney failure itself. I did this in the appendix and the review of the literature itself. It is difficult to understand what kidney failure can do to someone if we do not know what the normal kidney does. I wrote the appendix first, so that the project must be dealt with as a whole and the whole is greater than the sum of its parts, which is a phrase used to describe the kidney itself. One part of the project relates to the other parts and may be similar, but has certain differences.

My second problem was to help people cope with kidney failure. In order to do this, I did a thorough literature study on what kidney-failure patients had to cope with, including watching how a close friend handled kidney failure. I also reviewed suggestions from authors on how to cope with kidney failure. I feel that my friend on dialysis is a model of how to cope with kidney failure and dialysis. For one thing, if she has a problem, she voices it immediately, loudly and clearly. She turns dialysis into a chance to socialize and even a chance to sell for her business. She is trying to become successful at a business so that she can get off her disability pension. The advantage to being her own boss is that she does not have to work if she does not feel well, but she is making a strong effort to succeed in business. She cares about other people and has many friends that she has been very kind to. She seldom feels sorry for herself and bases her life on love, as well as courage. She lives on her own and does much of her own shopping with help from family and friends. She is religious and believes that God will reward her for good behaviour. She has confidence in most of her doctors and nurses and uses them to comfort her. She gets upset when someone on dialysis dies, probably because it reminds her of her own mortality. She bounces back from bad moods very quickly. Sometimes, she gets angry and I ask an hour later, "Are you still angry?" She says that she has forgotten all about it.

She likes to walk, but cannot walk very far because of her anemia, associated with kidney failure. She always does the best that she can.

Depression and anxiety are a major problem among kidney-failure patients. Depression can be helped by voicing your concerns, looking at the reason for the problem and finding a solution. Anxiety can be helped by learning to relax the muscles systematically. You get in touch with the slight tensions in various muscle groups, such as the wrist, forearm, arms, legs, back muscles, facial muscles, and eye muscles. Then you learn to let go of the tension after focusing on what the tension feels like and doing the opposite.

Vocational rehabilitation, finding what someone in kidney failure can and cannot do is very important. It is also important to deal with problems that may have nothing to do with kidney failure, such as low self-esteem, since problems like that will be multiplied and complicated by kidney failure.

The third problem that I felt needed to be addressed was for a patient with end-stage renal disease to have hope. My original goal was to study the kidney and the dialysis machine and try to build an implantable artificial kidney by extrapolating on them. After I looked at the dialysis machine, and the complex kidney, I was so discouraged that I wanted to do another project. Even the director of kidney transplants at Toronto Hospital, a nephrologist, said that an implantable kidney could not be made. With encouragement from Dr. Brownson and much research, I found that kidney failure was something on which I had much to offer. I came across researchers, Woods, Humes, Cieslinski, and Cutler who were working on a bioartificial kidney and had good success implanting it into animals. I felt that by making kidney patients aware of this tissue engineering technology and how relevant and highly developed it was, I could give kidney-failure patients hope. Also, the story of Willem Kolff's perseverance in developing a dialysis machine gave hope. There were a few other promising avenues of research, but I feel that the tissue-engineering approach of Humes is the most promising.

Results and Summary

One of the results of doing this work was a much greater compassion and understanding for someone who is going through kidney failure. Anger is a natural reaction for someone going through kidney failure and learning this caused me to stop criticising a man in dialysis who was always complaining about the nurses and the "poorly run" dialysis room. I realized that he was angry and I just said "it must be hard to be a dialysis patient." As more evidence that the rigors of kidney failure routine cause anger, my friend had two violence codes called on her in the course of just a few weeks. She had to have a large number of personnel and security officers surround her, even though I thought that she was not capable of violence. Indeed, her lack of coordination would be another factor that would prevent her from hurting someone.

I also learned never to give up. Willem Kolff, the inventor of dialysis had sixteen patients die before he saved the life of the seventeenth. Just when I thought that an implantable artificial kidney was impossible, I found that it indeed had been done successfully in small animals.

Another thing that I learned from the project was some of the medical problems facing kidney-failure patients. I feel that this work informs the public on these problems in a very useful way. I always translate technical terms into a common explanation, where possible.

The book that I wrote begins with the normal anatomy and physiology of the kidney. Included are feedback mechanisms and the importance of keeping these in balance. It describes the structure of the kidney and the nephron. We can see from this work just what kidney failure would do to someone.

Chapter 8 deals with causes of kidney failure and some important considerations in chronic renal failure are discussed. Diabetic nephropathy is the most common cause of kidney failure. Some important considerations in renal failure are: calcium metabolism derangement and red blood cell derangement. Kidney transplant as a form of treatment is dealt with here.

The book then goes into treatment of kidney failure, describing what a transplant entails and how to cope with it. The diet for a transplant is just a normal, healthy diet. Antirejection drugs are important and they are one of the down sides to a kidney transplant because of their side effects.

Chapter 9 deals with other treatments for ESRD, including the different forms of dialysis and some direction on how to do it so that the patient's family can know whether they want to be trained in it or not. It is not intended to be a manual on how to do dialysis, but to help people decide whether or not they want to do home dialysis. What to expect on dialysis is discussed, as well as vascular access and some of its problems. Diet of a dialysis patient is also a part of this chapter.

Chapter 10 deals with some psychological problems of a person in kidney failure. It shows kidney-failure patients that they are not alone in their situation. Suicidal ideation is dealt with as well as suicide in general. Some of the difficulties of kidney-failure patients and their spouses are discussed. Actual psychological disorders of ESRD patients are dealt with next. Adjustment to kidney failure and dialysis is next and how people cope with the decreased sexual function is discussed. Exercise for kidney patients is discussed next and how kidney patients must adjust to decreased ability to exercise, even though some people have run marathons with kidney failure. Finally, optimising long-term care of kidney-failure patients is discussed.

The eleventh and final chapter is on kidney failure research and the main aspect of this is how close David Humes is to developing a cure for kidney failure. There is a long description of how a bioartificial kidney would work and how it would be implanted into the iliac arteries and veins in the groin, the same as in a kidney transplant. The fifth chapter also focuses on how a bioartificial kidney would be made, why it is necessary and some important considerations to a bioartificial kidney.

I feel that this project was a big success. The first problem that it answers is what is happening to the kidney-failure patient's body and why they have to take certain medications. This question was handled by dealing with normal kidney anatomy and physiology first. Knowing normal anatomy and physiology of the kidney not only helps someone understand kidney failure and what it does to the body, but also helps us understand the bioartificial kidney and its functions.

The second problem was to discuss how to cope with kidney failure and I feel that this is discussed very well in the appendix and to a certain extent in the prerequisite chapter three. This problem is given very thorough treatment and meets its objective. The third problem that I discuss was hope for the future. In the final chapter of the appendix, I outline in detail why there will soon be a better treatment for end-stage renal disease. I am very pleased with this work.

One problem that I had in doing this project was difficulty obtaining information. I just had to be patient and persistent. I waited two months for the material on the bioartificial kidney to come from the University of Michigan.

Another problem that I had was making my work original. This was satisfied by the fact that the whole is greater than the sum of its parts, so that even though I borrowed heavily from other authors, I not only injected some of my own ideas but created something that is very different than anything I have ever seen.

I would not do much differently, but I would have contacted the University of Michigan earlier for their material on the bioartificial kidney so that I would not have to delay my project for so long.

<<<MISSING PAGE 40>>>

and that people should appreciate having functioning kidneys. I feel grateful every time I eat a high-potassium food or take a few cups of tea. The kidney has a long list of functions in addition to purifying the blood. I hope that this book can help patients and their families who want to know more about the physical and emotional side of kidney failure and why there is so much hope for the future.

Appendix

HOPE AND HELP FOR KIDNEY FAILURE

Kidney Failure and
Its Treatment

A discussion of kidney failure must begin with a discussion of the normal anatomy and physiology of the kidney. The functions of the kidney are two-fold. One function is the maintenance of a normal steady state of body fluids and functions. The other function is as a site for making and breaking down of essential body functions (Schnermann, 1998, p.1). Maintenance of the normal steady state of the body requires feedback mechanisms. This means that when variable A rises, variable B falls, or when variable A rises, variable B falls. The first process is called a positive feedback loop, and the second process (when variable A rises, variable B falls) is called a negative feedback loop. The end result is a maintenance of the body steady state called homeostasis.

For example, if substance A is a substance called renin, a hormone secreted by the kidney that helps to regulate blood pressure rises, substance B, angiotensin 2, a substance that raises blood pressure, rises. The net result is a rise in blood pressure. By the same token, if substance B rises (e.g. angiotensin 2 rises), substance A (renin) falls. The net result is a lowering of blood pressure because renin is a more powerful agent in raising blood pressure. The net result is to maintain blood pressure at its normal steady state where it should be (Schermann, 1998 p. 1). An odd number of negative feedback loops stabilises the body and an even number of positive feedback loops causes a rising of the substance or variable. This situation can be catastrophic for the body if the level of a substance rises too high or goes too low (Schermann, 1998 p. 2). The whole idea is for net gains to equal net losses. The kidneys are the organs involved in the control of electrolytes, water, metabolic end products, and foreign substances (Schnermann, 1998, p. 3). Examples of electrolytes are: sodium, potassium, phosphates, calcium, water, magnesium, and sulphates, or any other substance that conducts electricity. These substances are, in fact, called electrolytes because they conduct electricity. The kidneys also help to maintain hydrogen ion balance. In this way, they control the acid-base metabolism of the body. With ideal working of the kidneys, there is a steady state of metabolic end products, such as urea, uric acid, and creatinine (a waste product produced by muscles). In fact, creatinine levels in the blood are used to measure kidney function (Schermann, 1998, p. 4).

The kidneys also function as endocrine glands that secrete substances that have a biochemical effect on the body. Examples are: renin, which is an enzyme that breaks down angiotensin 2. Angiotensin 2 is a protein hormone that increases vascular tone and consequently increases blood pressure. Also, angiotensin 2 maintains fluid balance outside cells by affecting kidney absorption of sodium. The kidneys also secrete erythropoietin that stimulate production of red blood cells in the bone marrow. The kidneys also process vitamin D to its active form in calcitriol, which increases calcium in the blood. Calcitriol is also called 1,25-dihydroxyvitamin D3. Also, the kidneys produce glucose, angiotensinogen (the end product of renin) and ammonia. Because the kidneys break insulin, a kidney-failure patient needs less insulin (Schermann, 1998, pp. 6-7). In summary, kidneys regulate water and salt balance, potassium balance, blood pressure, red blood cell production in bone marrow and calcium metabolism metabolism metabolism. This shows what kidney failure can do to someone if these mechanisms are not working properly.

Kidney Structure

The inner middle side of the kidney has a deep indentation called the renal hilum. It is there that the kidney connects to blood and lymphatic vessels, nerves, and the ureters, structures that carry urine down to the bladder (Schnermann, 1998, p. 11). The bladder holds urine and sometimes excretes it, when it gets full, through the urethra.

In an up-and-down cross-section of the outward section of reddish-brown cortex of the kidney, it is different from a paler-striped inner region of the kidney called the medulla. The medulla is cone-shaped, and the base of the cone comes in contact with the cortex. The tip of the cone-shaped part of the kidney is the place where urine drains into a composite of the cortex and medulla, called the papilla. The urine drains from the papillae to the renal pelvis to the ureter, then from the bladder to the urethra (Schnermann, 1998, p. 11).

The kidney tissue consists of renal tubules and arteries entering the cortex. No arteries enter the renal medulla (Schnermann, 1998, p. 12). What enters the cortex is afferent arterioles (afferent means going in). They have a diameter of about 0.1 millimeters and form a vascular bed called the glomerulus. Glomeruli are only found in the cortex and drain into the efferent arterioles (efferent means leaving). The blood vessels supplying the medulla are derived from there (efferent arterioles). Lymph vessels are also found only in the cortex (Schnermann, 1998, pp. 12-13).

The kidney tissues consist of tubules that are lined by a single layer of cells. Tubules vary in length between four and eight centimeters. The functional unit of the kidney is called the nephron and consists of the glomerulus and its associated tubules. Each kidney contains about one million nephrons. The capsule of the kidney is closed and is called Bowman's capsule. It makes intimate contact with the capillaries of the glomerulus. Connected to the glomerulus are tubules. The closest one is called the proximal tubule which leads into the loop of Henle to the connecting duct and then the distal tubule. The urine then goes to the outer tubules and then the renal pelvis (Schnermann, 1998, pp. 14-15). As we shall see, this knowledge of the anatomy and physiology of the normal kidney is very important when constructing a bioartificial kidney.

Urine Formation

The formation of urine, which is the excretory product of the kidneys, proceeds in two sequential, but different steps. They are: glomerular ultrafiltration, which just means filtering out waste products by the glomeruli, and tubular absorption and secretion (Schnermann, 1998, p. 19). Absorption is defined as the movement of solutes or water from the tubular lumen (middle) to the blood, regardless of the mechanism. It can occur through the cells or between the cells.

Absorption (or reabsorption) is the main process in the renal handling of sodium, chloride, water, bicarbonate, glucose, amino acids, proteins, phosphates, calcium, magnesium, and other substances (Schnermann, 1998, p. 20).

Secretion is defined as the movement of solutes from blood to tubular lumen to urine. It is important in the renal handling of hydrogen ions, which help regulate the acid-base composition of the blood, potassium, ammonia, and others (Schnermann, 1998, p. 20).

The above information was corroborated by Stewart Cameron (1996). He said that the normal function of the kidney is to eliminate wastes, water, and to produce hormones to regulate blood pressure, red blood cell formation, and calcium metabolism (Cameron, 1996, p.4; Ganong, 1995, p. 641). The kidneys regulate water metabolism by excreting the excess as urine. They regulate blood pressure by excreting excess fluid and producing a hormone called renin, which elevates the blood pressure. They also cause production of angiotensin 2, which also raises the blood pressure. They regulate calcium metabolism by secreting calcitriol, a hormone that raises blood calcium. They regulate red blood cell production by secreting erythropoietin-releasing factor that encourages the bone marrow to produce more red blood cells (Ganong, 1995, p. 641).

Cameron also concurs that each kidney is not a single organ, but is made up of about one million units called nephrons. The word, nephron comes from the Greek word for kidney, "nephros." The Latin word for kidney is "renes," so that a number of words pertaining to the kidney are from those roots, such as renal failure and nephritis, the former meaning kidney failure and the latter meaning kidney inflammation (Cameron, 1996, p. 4).

Some of the functions of the nephron are completed in the outer surface of the kidney called the cortex, mainly the glomerulus. The glomerulus is a bunch of capillaries with thin walls to allow it to act as a filter. The tubules lead from the cortex and glomeruli to the inner portion of the kidney, the medulla. The fluid going back into circulation comes up the other side of the tubule to concentrate it and the waste products pass into the ureters and then the bladder for excretion (Cameron, 1998, pp. 5-7). The tubules run in parallel through the medulla and are also called the loop of Henle.

How Kidneys Work

One of the most important units of the nephron is the glomerulus. It takes in blood under pressure and filters off about one fifth of the water in the blood with its dissolved salts. Water and dissolved salts are smaller molecules than protein and other cells that normal kidneys do not let through. Therefore, protein in the urine (especially albumen) is a frequent indicator of kidney disease (Cameron, 1996, p. 8). It is especially common in Bright's disease. The kidneys process about 50 gallons of water each day and the body contains about twelve gallons. Therefore, the kidneys process all the water in the body about four times per day. About 99.5% of salts and water are reabsorbed into the bloodstream and three to five pints of urine are passed off from the bladder (Cameron, 1996, p. 9). Among the functions of the kidney are: filtering out poisons, such as urea, maintaining a balance between sodium chloride (table salt) and water, regulation of body fluid balance, regulation of potassium balance, and regulation of a balance between sodium and potassium ions.

It also functions to maintain a proper balance of glucose, amino acids, bile salts, and other organic (carbon-based) charged particles. The function of the kidneys in maintaining calcium and phosphate balance is crucial. The balance of these chemicals is critical for muscle and bone function and is important to maintain acid-base balance of the body. A person cannot live without adequate calcium and phosphate balance and proper acid-base balance. The kidneys excrete hydrogen ions, which as mentioned, directly helps maintain acid-base balance of the body. Someone in kidney failure needs a dialysis machine to perform some of these functions and medications such as calcium carbonate and calcitriol to do the rest. One of the signs of acid blood is faster and deeper breathing because hydrogen ions stimulate the respiratory centre in the brain (Schnermann, 1998, pp. 1-201).

The nephron is essentially made of blood vessel type cells, which is why a bioartificial kidney can be made from blood vessel type cells, especially the person's own cells, in order to override the problem of rejection. Cells coming from the same person are not foreign and therefore will not be attacked. Another alternative to using the patient's own cells, in order to override the problem of rejection is to encapsulate the foreign cells with a substance that acts as a buffer between the foreign cells and the cells of the body (Cutler, 1999). The nephron is the functional unit of the kidney, but because of the way the nephrons function together, a kidney is more than just a collection of one million nephrons (Ganong, 1995, p. 643).

There are many holes in many parts of the nephron to allow fluids and substances to pass in and out. The tubules and the nephron are so small and so complex, that it is almost impossible to duplicate kidney function exactly. In order to make a bioartificial kidney, we must borrow some of the function of an outside of the body artificial kidney, the dialysis machine. That is what David Humes and John Woods have tried to do.

While a nephron is very tiny in diameter, it is very long. It is approximately 14 mm in length, including the tubules (Ganong, 1995, p. 644). That is primarily what makes the kidney so large (it is the size of a fist) and makes it more feasible to duplicate the function. It is the thinness of the nephron that is difficult to duplicate. However, as can be seen from dialysis machines, a bioartificial kidney does not have to exactly duplicate a real kidney.

Kidney Circulation

The kidneys really are remarkable organs. They process 1.2-1.3 litres of blood per minute, which is close to 25% of total cardiac output. As mentioned, this amounts to 10-12 gallons a day or four times our total blood volume (Ganong, 1995, p. 645). This concurs with Schnermann's account of kidney function, but in more detail. A high-protein diet raises the pressure in the kidney and increases kidney blood flow. It is very important to maintain an appropriate amount of pressure in the kidneys. Too much pressure can damage the kidneys and too little pressure can cause lack of circulation through the kidneys, also causing damage (Ganong, 1995, p. 540). In fact, there is speculation that diabetic nephropathy damages the kidneys by decreasing the pressure inside them and stagnating the blood (Ganong, 1995, p. 646). However, other authors feel that it is deposition of glycosylated end-products from diabetes that damages the kidney (McPhee, 1997, p. 381). Nobody knows for sure.

In the kidney, there is a countercurrent mechanism for concentrating urine, which simply means that the urine passes through the loop of Henle twice to concentrate the urine. It does so in a parallel way (Ganong, 1995, p. 657).

Role of Urea

Urea is a waste product produced by breakdown of protein in the liver. It is then passed on through the bloodstream to the kidneys for excretion. It helps to concentrate urine. Some people used to say that a low-protein diet is best for failing kidneys because it makes less work for them (Ganong, 1995, p.658). Now some people say that a high protein diet is good for kidney failure to make someone strong enough to fight off the disease and prevent wasting of tissues (Patterson, 1996).

People in kidney failure have to watch their fluid intake because excess fluid can overload the heart, for one thing. Also, it can cause swelling of brain cells due to water intoxication, which is deadly (Ganong, 1995, p.659). It is blood urea nitrogen (BUN) and creatinine that determine the severity of kidney failure. BUN is a waste product of digestion caused by breakdown of protein in the liver, and creatinine is a waste product of muscle contraction (Ganong, 1995, p. 666). In previous days, uremia—or kidney failure—was simply described as a rising of the BUN, but this has changed because BUN is affected greatly by diet. Now, creatinine clearance is the indicator of kidney function. This will be discussed in relation to kidney transplants later on.

When the kidneys do not do their job properly, urea and creatinine accumulate in the blood. There is lethargy (tiredness), loss of appetite, nausea, vomiting, mental deterioration and confusion, muscle twitching, convulsions, and eventually coma and death. Some people argue that it is the accumulation of toxic substances other than urea and creatinine, like phenols and organic acids, that cause the deadly symptoms of kidney failure, but no one is certain (Ganong, 1995, p. 667).

McPhee believes that the fatigue and malaise caused by kidney failure are the result of the loss of the ability of the kidney to excrete water, salt, and wastes via the kidneys. Later on, the brain can malfunction due to excess toxins (McPhee, 1997, p. 383).

Causes of Chronic
Renal Failure

McPhee lists the most common cause of renal failure as diabetes mellitus. High blood pressure and inflammation of the kidney closely follow diabetes mellitus as causes of chronic renal failure. Because of damage to the kidneys, a greater functional burden is borne by fewer nephrons, which causes increased pressure inside the nephron and scars it in a process called "sclerosis." (McPhee, 1997, p. 386). Diabetic nephropathy is sometimes called capillary glomerulosclerosis or Kimmelstiel-Wilson's disease (Gilmore, 1995).

Important Considerations in Chronic Renal Failure

Sometimes sodium bicarbonate is given during the early stages of chronic renal failure in order to combat the acid blood caused by an inability to excrete hydrogen ions. Later on, dialysis removes hydrogen ions (Cole, 1994).

It is also important to note that much phosphate competes with calcium and leads to a lack of calcium, which can cause a weakness of bones and fractures as well as malfunction of the parathyroid glands that regulate calcium metabolism and can cause muscle and nerve damage (McPhee, 1997, p.388). Accordingly, a calcium-producing and phosphate-binding substance called calcium carbonate is given in order to normalise the function. It is very effective. Stomach ulcers are also a result of this calcium deficiency, although the mechanism is not clear (McPhee, 1997, p. 389).

Also, bleeding, bruising, and blood abnormalities due to lack of erythropoietin— as mentioned—characterises chronic renal failure. The toxins produced by kidney failure tend to suppress white blood cells so that there is a decreased ability to fight off infections. This makes it important for kidney patients to get influenza vaccines, pneumonia vaccines, and hepatitis B vaccines (Cole, 1996).

The book *Nephrology* by Craig Fisher and Christopher Wilcox corroborated what was said above and had nothing to add to the discussion of chronic renal failure.

A person can survive with as little as 3-5% of his kidney function. This gives a great deal of reserve in case of temporary kidney malfunction, but a person in chronic renal failure does not even have 3-5% of their kidney function (Cameron, 1996, p. 3).

Kidney-failure patients lose the ability to urinate. This constitutes the loss of a body function. Losing a body function such as urination is similar to losing a limb and causes a grieving process. My friend on dialysis says that she finds it very frustrating not to be able to urinate. It is important to know how to help people cope with this problem. My friend is basically a happy person and copes very well. Others do not cope so well and get belligerent or resentful. I have seen this on the dialysis floor. By listening to a patient's frustrations and showing empathy, it can greatly reduce someone's frustration. Empathy is a matter of being able to imagine how the other person feels without losing your own identity.

Treatment of Kidney Failure

The choices to patients regarding treatment are hemodialysis, continuous ambulatory peritoneal dialysis (CAPD), continuous cycling peritoneal dialysis (CCPD), and kidney transplant. The advantage to a kidney transplant is increased hope and not being tied to dialysis. The disadvantages to kidney transplant are the numerous side effects of the antirejection drugs, especially impairment of the immune system's function. This impairment of the immune system's function can cause infections and cancer risk.

Kidney Transplant: An Option for Kidney Patients

The members of the kidney transplant team include transplant nephrologists, kidney doctors who specialise in kidney transplantation problems, the kidney transplant surgeon and his team, the transplant coordinator who tells people what receiving a kidney transplant entails and coordinates the program and who is usually a registered nurse, the transplant social worker who helps patients with the logistics of problems related to a kidney transplant such as where they will live and who will look after them, a registered dietitian, a psychiatrist and psychiatric nurse, a general physician, and a general registered nurse.

There are approximately eighty different kidney diseases, and diabetic nephropathy is the one that most commonly causes kidney failure.

Although dialysis is a lifesaving treatment, it cannot perform the functions of real kidneys. This is one reason why a kidney transplant offers more advantages than dialysis. The doctor can recommend what is best for you.

There are preconditions for a person to meet before he or she undergoes a transplant:

(1)   A patient must be physically fit for having a transplant and understand the risks and benefits of a transplant as well as responsibilities after a transplant.
(2)   You must complete an assessment that shows you can benefit from the transplant and tolerate an anesthetic and surgery and do not have any other active medical problems.
(3)   You must be free of active infection.
(4)   You must not have active cancer or be receiving chemotherapy for cancer.

Kidney transplant is a treatment for kidney failure, but not a cure. The average life span of a kidney coming from a brain-dead person is eight to ten years. Living person donations last longer. You must believe that the advantages outweigh the disadvantages.

Among the advantages are:

(1)   Freedom from dialysis.
(2)   Increased energy.
(3)   Less restricted diet and no fluid restrictions.
(4)   Increased hemoglobin, meaning more exercise tolerance because there is more hemoglobin to carry oxygen to cells.
(5)   Increased feeling of well-being. (McKnight, 1997, p. 5).

Among the disadvantages are:

(1)   Taking antirejection drugs for the rest of your life.

(2)   Required follow-up at the transplant clinic for life. At first, this is four times per week for several months, but after about a year, it decreases to once a week and later once a month.

(3)   The side effects of antirejection medications, which can be quite frightening. For example antirejection drugs weaken the immune system and make you more vulnerable to infection and certain cancers. This can be ameliorated by checking for the warning signs of cancer and checking the skin. Also, if you have a psychosis, prednisone—an antirejection drug—will aggravate this, possibly severely. Prednisone can cause confusion and loss of memory. The warning signs of cancer are: sores that do not heal, change in appearance of a wart or mole, change in bowel or bladder habits, difficulty swallowing, coughing up blood, persistent vomiting or loss of appetite, and loss of weight, or pain without explanation. In addition to increased risk of cancer, antirejection drugs can cause diabetes or elevate someone from non-insulin dependent diabetes to insulin-dependent diabetes, and cause weight gain from a ravenous appetite. Diet and exercise can combat this (Cotter, 1998).

(4)   Another disadvantage to kidney transplant is the stress of worrying about the kidney failing. The success rate for kidney transplants is 85% for the first year, but there is a steady decline after that.

A pretransplant evaluation must be done. This includes a chest X-ray, electrocardiogram, and two-dimensional echocardiogram. Also, a persantine thallium scan to assess circulation to the heart must be done. Barium swallows and gastroscopy must be done to satisfy that stomach trouble will not interfere with the transplant procedure (McKnight, 1997, p. 11)

Other procedures that must be done are cystoscopy to make sure the bladder is fit to receive a kidney transplant; blood typing of A, B, O, Rh; and genetic typing. Type AB blood can receive a kidney from anyone. Types O, A, and B can only receive blood from their own blood type—with the exception of types A and B, who can receive blood and kidneys from type O as well as their own blood type. The circulation of blood to the pelvic area must be tested in order to make sure that the pelvic artery can handle a transplant.

Cytotoxic antibody studies must be done for tissue matching. For example, if someone donates a kidney that is a perfect match for someone's tissue type, that person (recipient) would receive preference in obtaining a kidney transplant. The transplant team tries to match tissue types as well as possible so that there is the least chance of rejection. The transplant team must also be sure that both parties are free of infections, such as hepatitis B or C or HIV.

Waiting for a Transplant

The process of waiting for a transplant can range from a few months to several years and can involve much anxiety and disappointment. Patients on the waiting for a kidney transplant carry beepers that can go off any time of the day or night. The average wait is three to five years. With type A blood, because it is more common, three and a half years is an expected waiting period. However, many factors are taken into account, including degree of tissue match, as mentioned, and availability of dialysis. If someone has difficulty getting dialysis, he will be higher on the list. The beeper can go off within a few months if an exact match is found and patients are advised to have a plan already in place in case the beeper goes off at an unexpected time. It can go off at three in the morning or twelve noon or anytime (Cotter, 1998).

Matching the Donor with the Recipient

This process is based on a number of factors. One is blood type. In order to receive a donor kidney, the recipient's blood must be compatible with the donor's blood as was mentioned earlier. Tissue typing and genetic typing are also used in matching the donor with the recipient. Cadaveric (dead) donors are more difficult to match, which means that antirejection drugs are that much more important. There are a series of six significant areas on the chromosomes (the containers of genetic material) that should match up between donor and recipient. A relative acting as a live donor can usually match three of these factors and sometimes more. An identical twin would be perfect. There are also some areas of cross-matching that are not known yet. Dead donors usually do not match genetic typing at all. Cytotoxic antibodies are tested with the recipient by mixing donor blood with patient blood. No reaction (negative) means that the match is good. A positive test means that there are antibodies in your blood or his blood and the transplant cannot proceed.

For those receiving a cadaveric (dead person's) kidney, the considerations are, as mentioned: blood and tissue cross-match, access to dialysis, and length of wait for a transplant. Part of getting a kidney is the luck of the draw. A province wide computer (multiple organ retrieval and exchange, or MORE) holds all the data about transplants, and if you are fit for a transplant, your name is added to the list (McKnight, 1997, p. 14).

Advice to People Waiting for a Transplant

(1)   Live life to the fullest. Do not aggravate yourself by waiting for the beeper to go off. However, keep the transplant team apprised of your whereabouts at all times in case they need to reach you.

(2)   Stay as healthy as possible while you wait. Exercise, if possible, even if all you can manage are short walks. Eat a good diet, following your dietitian's plan. Try to reduce being overweight as this increases surgical risks.

(3)   Let the dialysis team know if you have a minor illness such as a cold or flu so the transplant will be put off temporarily or held if it comes up.

Call your transplant coordinator if you have any concerns. Also, counseling may be necessary to help you work out your feelings from a false alarm. False alarms can come from many sources. For example, the kidney may be found to be unsuitable after testing, or you may see a doctor walking toward you grim-faced and telling you that the kidney deteriorated in transit.

Kidney transplants are by far the most frequent of all transplants in Toronto, with about one hundred being performed each year. There are five hundred people on the waiting list.

When you get your call from the transplant center, you will feel excitement and fear that can cloud the mind. You must have a definitive plan in place that will allow you to take definitive action if necessary. This cannot be stressed enough. You must get to the hospital and not eat or drink anything after your call. Also, only one to two hours is the waiting time after contacting you. After that, another recipient will be selected.

The incision is approximately eight to ten inches in length in the right or left lower abdomen. The new kidney is attached to the iliac arteries in the pelvis, and the ureters are reattached to the bladder. The nonfunctioning kidneys are left in place. The surgery usually takes two to three hours. The surgeon attaches the artery and vein of your new kidney to the artery and vein going to your leg. A bladder catheter is inserted to drain urine and a jugular line is put into the neck to give fluids and medications. They may put in an endotracheal tube in the throat to assist breathing as the anesthetic slows the breathing process and the anesthetic may impair your ability to breathe on your own. Pain medication is given as needed. Once awake, the doctor will give you a pain pump so that you can give yourself pain medication. This is attached to your body and is more effective because you can give yourself pain medication when you feel a need for it.

Kidney scans, ultrasound, and simple leg exercises are done. The intensive care unit staff will help you get up as soon as possible.

The main health issues are monitoring for rejection, adjusting immunosuppressive therapy, education, rehabilitation, and reassurance.

Deep breathing and coughing are important postoperatively to ensure functioning of the respiratory system and to prevent accumulation of fluids and secretions in the lungs.

Weight gain is also important to watch. It may show fluid retention, which is a sign of rejection. Chest X-rays, abdominal and pelvic ultrasound, two-dimensional echocardiograms, and teaching on what to expect are done.

Exercise is an important part of therapy to increase muscle tone, increase appetite, and prevent the complications due to inactivity such as fecal impaction or bowel obstruction, kidney stasis, heart weakness, atherosclerosis, deep vein thrombosis, and a few other complications.

Among the complications of a kidney transplant are rejection, infection, antetubular necrosis, and obstruction. Antetubular necrosis means dying of the kidney tubules that are involved in reabsorption of substances, and obstruction of these tubules can also occur. Obstruction of the tubules refers to anything that gets in the way of normal kidney function. Any unusual symptoms should be reported immediately. Rejection occurs when the body's immune system attacks the kidney, which is seen as foreign tissue. Also, the kidney can attack the patient's cells, which is called graft versus host disease. Infection is always a problem with surgery.

Signs of rejection are:

(1) fever.
(2) pain in the kidney.
(3) fluid retention, such as shown by increased blood pressure.

(4)   increased weight.
(5)   decreased urine output, meaning that the kidney is not functioning as it should.
(6)   edema, caused by an inability to excrete water so that fluid builds up in tissues and the lungs. When fluid builds up in the lungs, it is a medical emergency.
(7)   flulike symptoms and sniffles.

Signs of infection are fever, chills, cough, pain on voiding, and drainage of pus (McKnight, 1997, p. 35).

Acute tubular necrosis is due to moving one kidney to another person. It is also referred to as sleepy kidney. It literally means "dying of the tubules," and hemodialysis may be necessary. For obstruction, a tube must be inserted (Cotter, 1998).

After surgery, the immunosuppressive drugs can make you tired, confused, disoriented, unable to concentrate, and unable to sleep. Sometimes medications are needed to counteract these side effects.

With kidney transplantation, there are some effects such as increased appetite leading to weight gain, increased blood pressure, increased blood fat and cholesterol levels, and increased blood sugar. These are usually related to transplant medications, fewer food restrictions, increased blood sugar, and increased feeling of well-being. You must therefore control salt, fat, and cholesterol in diet. It is recommended that you walk one to five minutes, six to nine times daily. Increase this by one minute per day per week as tolerated. When you are up to fifteen minutes at one time, increase speed.

Lower Fat and Lower Cholesterol Tips

(1)   Choose lean meats, fish, and poultry.
(2)   Choose low-fat milk and dairy products.
(3)   Bake, broil, steam, and poach foods. Do not fry them.
(4)   Avoid palm oil, hydrogenated vegetable oils, and shortening as these contain saturated fat.
(5)   Avoid luncheon meats, wieners, and fast foods.
(6)   Use small amounts of polyunsaturated/monounsaturated fats that tend to lower blood cholesterol such as corn oil, sunflower oil, canola oil, soya oil, and olive oils. Use soft margarine.
(7)   Check labels for fat and cholesterol.
(8)   Avoid high-cholesterol foods like egg yolks, shrimp, and organ meats.

Healthy Weight Tips

(1) Eat three regular meals per day, breakfast included.
(2) Decrease serving size.
(3) Decrease high-calorie, fat-laden foods.
(4) Eat slowly and stop when full.
(5) Choose nutritious low-calorie snacks like fruits and vegetables to satisfy your appetite.
(6) Shop on a full stomach to avoid impulse buying of bad foods.
(7) Choose foods from the four foods groups: grains, ??? and vegetables, milk and dairy products, and meat and legumes ??? other protein foods.

Antirejection Drugs

These drugs help treat and prevent rejection of the new ??? well as protect the body from graft versus host disease as men ??? earlier.

The first drug group is anti lymphocyte drugs, such as a ??? thymocyte serum. OKT3 is an example of this. It is only given ??? hospital.

Another important drug to suppress the immune system is ??? prednisone. It is also anti-inflammatory. Some of its side effects are stomach irritation, fluid retention, facial puffiness, increased appe???, increased blood sugar, increased susceptibility to infection, increased hair growth, acne, cataracts, and menstrual irregularities. It is recommended that kidney patients carry a medic alert bracelet.

Another antirejection drug is cyclosporine. Its side effects are: increased blood pressure, making hands tremble, making gums swell, stomach upset, nausea and loss of appetite, susceptibility to infection, and increased risk of cancer. Cyclosporine can also be toxic to the kidney.

Another antirejection drug is azothiopurine. It suppresses the immune system as does cyclosporine. Among its side effects are stomach upset, dark urine, yellow skin, lower hemoglobin, bruising and bleeding, susceptibility to infection, and increased risk of cancer.

The last antirejection drug that I will mention is mycophenolate. It inhibits the function of white blood cells to attack the transplanted organ. Among its adverse effects are stomach upset, increased chance of infection, and increased risk of cancer.

As can be seen, although there are certain advantages to kidney transplant—such as freedom, not needing dialysis, and feeling better—there are some disadvantages, such as having to take antirejection drugs with their side effects.

This section on kidney transplant was taken from (Teresa McKnight and Brenda McQuaine, *Kidney Transplant Manual*, The Toronto Hospital publishing, Multi Organ Transplant Program, 1997).

McGee and Bradley state that weakening of the immune system and increased susceptibility to cancer are common concerns with end-stage renal disease patients (McGee and Bradley, 1994, p. 8). I found this to be very frightening in a meeting with Lorna Cotter, the transplant coordinator at Toronto Hospital. My friend was as frightened as I was.

Other Treatments for Kidney Failure and Coping with Kidney Failure

Currently, the treatment for kidney failure—other than kidney transplant—is dialysis in its different forms. Hemodialysis involves pumping blood around a circuit outside the body in which is placed a filter or "dialyser." There is a bundle of hemodialysis row fibers through which the blood flows, everything being contained in a plastic container through which a carefully prepared salt solution or "dialysate" is flushed in order to cleanse the fibers. Waste products diffuse through the walls of the fibres to the "dialysing" fluid, which is discarded. The dialysate returns materials to the blood and supplies a buffer to neutralise metabolic acids derived from protein breakdown. The process requires a somewhat complicated monitor and machine and highly purified water to produce large volumes of dialysate. It is usually performed in a hospital, but when patients are highly motivated and have a trainable partner, it can be performed in the home (McGee and Bradley, 1994, pp. 15-16).

John Sedgewick states that enabling patients and family members to assume a self-care role is important. Not all patients are capable of a self-care role, but it tends to make them feel more empowered (1998, pp. 45-46).

One of the most effective forms of self-care is peritoneal dialysis, particularly tidal peritoneal dialysis. It maintains a high dose of dialysis by maintaining a combination of constant and intermittent flow in the abdominal cavity. It only drains off part of the fluid at a time, hence the name "tidal peritoneal dialysis." Peritoneal dialysis consists of having the doctor insert a catheter into the abdomen and having the patient fill this catheter with fluid at certain specified times and then drain the water off at other specified times. It is best to follow the instructions of a therapist to know exactly how to do home dialysis, but I will attempt to describe the process, eventually. Complications of peritoneal dialysis consist of infection, distorted body image, herniated bowels and damage to internal organs (Sedgewick, 1998, p. 154).

Charlene Reeves, in her book on medical-surgical nursing said that dialysis (hemodialysis) consists of filtering fluid from the blood and putting it through an external dialysis machine, containing a coil that acts as a semipermeable membrane (1999, p. 225). The three stages of dialysis are diminished reserve, renal insufficiency, and end-stage renal disease (ESRD).

Erythropoietin (EPO) and muscle cramps, seizures and abnormal reflexes are sometimes side effects of hemodialysis. Also, kidney failure causes dying of white blood cells, which is the main cause of death among dialysis patients (infection). Therefore, it is important to use strict aseptic technique (Reeves, 1999, p. 224). Edema, pain, redness, loss of appetite, low white blood cell count, malaise, and fatigue should be reported at once. Kussmaul's respirations—which are faster and deeper, more laboured breathing—are usually a sign of acid blood. This is dangerous. Patients should restrict fluid, phosphates, and protein intake.

First, in looking after a fistula for vascular access, feel for vibrations called thrills (do not tell someone that you are feeling for a thrill); listen for bruits, which are the tapping sounds made by a narrowing fistula; and apply no restrictive dressing to a narrow artery. This means no intravenous, no blood pressure, or taking blood on the side affected by the fistula.

Chronic leg cramps are a problem with dialysis. My friend gets this and sometimes the machine must be turned off to stop them. They can also be treated by stretching the leg muscles, moist, hot packs and massage. Blood pressure and pulse rate should be taken every half hour. Sodium and quinine sulphate also help get rid of leg cramps (Reeves, 1999, p. 225).

Sometimes there is headache, which is caused by urea being removed from the body faster than it is removed from the brain. This is called disequilibrium syndrome (Reeves, 1999, p. 226).

Patients should be weighed before and after dialysis. One needle goes into one end of the site, and another needle goes out. Expect weight loss with dialysis. When you take the patient off dialysis, stop the machine and hold the site with gauze there. Hold the site with gauze before removing the needle, and press until all bleeding stops (Reeves, 1999, p. 226).

Peritoneal dialysis is hard to do with obese or infected patients. You should weigh patients before each procedure. The peritoneum is perfused with dialysate fluid (Reeves, 1999, p. 226). This is done for ten to twenty minutes. It is left there for thirty to forty-five minutes. The dialysate should be sterilised with infrared and ultraviolet light. Then lower the waste product bag below the body and drain it. The doctor should figure out how often each day this should be done. The waste product should be pale yellow. At first, it can be bloody, but after the catheter is established, this is abnormal and should be reported. If the waste product dialysate fluid is cloudy, it may be a sign of infection. Vital signs should be taken, and the doctor should be notified. If the dialysate for peritoneal dialysis is brown, it may indicate a bowel perforation. The doctor should be informed immediately. Peritoneal dialysis can cause the loss of much protein, so the patient may need supplements (Reeves, 1999, p. 228).

In hemodialysis, there are four compartments. One is the blood compartment through which blood passes. Second is the dialysate compartment through which blood mixes with dialysate and passes through a semipermeable membrane separating blood from dialysate with cellulose derivatives. Third are the support structures for dialysis, and fourth are the small capillary-like tubes through which the blood passes. These are made from cellulose and synthetic membranes. Cellophane was the first one used (Sedgewick, 1998, pp. 98-99).

Heparin should be used to prevent clotting in the machine. It should not be used if the patient is bleeding heavily. If surgery was done up to five days before, the patient may bleed. If she moves too much, she may bleed. Much blood is transferred in a short space of time with hemodialysis. Also, if the patient is menstruating, heparin should be used lightly or not at all.

Alkalinity or acidity of the blood should be assessed. If the blood is acid, sodium bicarbonate should be given. Acetate is sometimes given as well. Water may also need to be given. These are added to the dialysis fluid. The arteriovenous fistula rate of success after three years is 56%-75%. There is much difficulty with this, and my friend has had different fistulas declotted several times.

I will now describe how to do home hemodialysis. Your nurse-educator should be the ultimate authority, and special training to do dialysis at home is important. The project will now discuss some of the procedures that someone on dialysis may have to go through, including a rough idea of how to do dialysis so that you know whether or not you want to go through home dialysis.

Femoral Catheters

These wide-bore femoral catheters have been very helpful to some people. Their wide bore enables a high rate of blood flow for dialysis. Femoral catheters are inserted under strict aseptic technique with the patient's head and feet raised. Local anesthesia is given, the femoral vein is punctured (cannulated), and the femoral catheter is inserted. The doctor must be careful not to spear the femoral artery. It is like being gored by a bull. The main worry about femoral catheterisation is infection. Bleeding from a femoral catheter is also a problem. The femoral catheter has an inflatable bulb in it so that it cannot come out.

One contraindication to femoral catheterisation is groin surgery because there is risk of bleeding. Femoral catheters are inserted only as a last resort. It is preferable to use the subclavian vein (in the shoulder) or an upper-body vein. In women, mammary veins have been used. Femoral veins are the worst place to have catheters put in because the area is dirty and this increases the risk of infection. Patients with femoral catheters usually cannot walk more than a few steps (Sedgewick, 1998, p. 114).

Arteriovenous Shunts

Shunts use special materials to join an artery with a vein, which is the original goal of vascular access anyway. There is a surgical cut-down and a joining of an artery and a vein with a Teflon-Silastic loop. The arteries and veins typically used are in the wrists or ankles. There are so many problems with this technique that it is rarely done.

Subclavian catheters are done more often and are placed in the shoulder. An X-ray is taken to make sure that the catheter was inserted properly. Strict hygiene is observed by the health care team and the patient because infection is a major worry (Sedgewick, 1998, p. 115).

Cannulation of an Arteriovenous Fistula

Before dialysis can be done, the fistula must have two needles in it. One brings blood out to the dialysis machine, and the other needle brings it back. Sticking the needles in is called cannulation.

First, a thorough assessment of the fistula must be done. The anatomy, vein length, and surgical formation must be known. There must be correct needle placement and correct choice of needle. The larger the bore of the needle, the more blood can be processed at once. However, too large a needle can damage the fistula. Patients with smaller veins need smaller needles (Sedgewick, 1998, p. 119).

Blood-flow direction within the arteriovenous fistula is the main factor influencing needle placement. The venous needle is placed in the direction of the venous return towards the heart, whereas the arterial needle is placed farther away from the heart. Hemodialysis can even be done with only one needle, with the one needle taking blood in and out (Sedgewick, 1998, p. 120). This one-needle dialysis is rare, and I have never seen it. Needles should be rotated to increase the lifespan of the arteriovenous fistula. Needle site rotation should be documented so that the caregiver knows where to place the needle the next time. If needles are placed all along the fistula, it will develop toughness and last longer (Sedgewick, 1998, p. 120).

The two best techniques for cannulation of a vascular access site are the rope ladder technique and the buttonhole technique. The rope ladder technique involves equal distribution of needle sites along the length of the vessel, causing uniform dilation of the vein with little or no clotting. The vessel is punctured on alternate sides during repeated dialysis (Sedgewick, 1998, p. 121).

The buttonhole technique involves using one to three sites for arterial and venous needles. The needle puncture at the same site and same angles builds up scar tissue so that needle placement does not hurt the patient. Using the same sites for puncture all the time promotes clotting and breakdown of the arteriovenous fistula.

Skin cleansing in order to prevent infection is essential to dialysis (Sedgwick, 1998, p. 123). Patients should be encouraged to wash the area of the needle placement, usually with a bactericidal soap. Then an antiseptic agent, possibly Betadine, should be applied. Gloves and goggles should ideally be worn by the caregiver, but I have seldom seen goggles used. The rationale behind goggles is not to have blood splash up into the caregiver's eyes (Sedgewick 1998, p. 123).

Local anaesthetics such as lidocaine can help reduce a patient's pain. This is important because the patient is more likely to comply with dialysis if it hurts less (Sedgewick, 1998, p. 123). Anytime you put a needle into someone, you set the clotting mechanism in motion, and this often leads to breakdown of the arteriovenous fistula, particularly if the patient has small veins.

Downward placement of needles causes less pain, according to studies done by Crespo (Sedgewick, 1998, p. 124). The needle should be held at a 45-degree angle for grafts and a 25—to 30-degree angle for arteriovenous fistulas. Once in the fistula, the needle should be inserted no further than 3 mm and then rotated 180 degrees (Sedgewick, 1998, p. 124). The needle should be secured with butterfly tape, a special type of tape with two wings. The more the needle moves, the less efficient the dialysis and the more damage it causes (Sedgewick, 1998, p. 124). If the needle punctures the vessel and comes into contact with the skin, it should be removed, hand pressure should be applied to the site, and the needle should be inserted somewhere else in the fistula. Heparin should only be used in the machine if needle placement is successful. Heparin prevents clotting of blood in the machine and is used for this purpose because it does not travel very much beyond the machine. As mentioned, it usually is not used if the patient is bleeding (as in menstruation) because some heparin does affect the patient somewhat.

At the end of dialysis, the needles should be removed gently so as not to damage the arteriovenous fistula. Pressure should be applied to the site to make sure bleeding is stopped. After that, a sterile dressing is applied, and the patient is weighed and can go wherever he or she wants to go. Clotting is the most common cause of failure of an arteriovenous fistula and infection is the second. It can be managed with aseptic techniques and antibiotic creams. Serious infections may require antibiotics by mouth (Sedgewick, 1998, p. 125).

Ischemia (lack of blood supply) near the vascular access site can lead to dying of tissue. I saw a patient with black, dead fingers from this "arterial steal" syndrome, in which flow through the fistula takes blood from surrounding tissues (Sedgewick, 1998, p. 126). He had to have some of his fingers removed.

Complications of vascular access for hemodialysis present the major cause of death among ESRD patients (Sedgewick, 1998, p. 132). Declotting with balloon angioplasty has an 84% success rate. This procedure involves inserting a tube inside the clotted arteriovenous fistula and pushing the clot into the artery or vein. It is so painful that Demerol, a strong narcotic painkiller, must be given to enable the patient to withstand the procedure. My friend has had it done several times.

The home dialysis machine is user-friendly so that, with a certain amount of training, patients can learn to do their own dialysis or have their partners do it. I included this section so that people would know whether or not they would want to do home dialysis.

Diet for Dialysis Patients

Most kidney patients on dialysis can only eat two high-potassium fruits or vegetables per day because they cannot excrete potassium. An excess of potassium stops in diastole (when the heart is relaxed) and is very dangerous. A lack of potassium, by contrast, stops the heart during systole (when the heart is contracted). Potassium is used to kill inmates who are sentenced to die by lethal injection. Also, most dialysis patients cannot have a healthy diet of grains and legumes because they contain too much potassium and phosphates. This further lowers the quality and quantity of life of a kidney patient. That is another reason why kidney failure needs new and better treatments (Patterson, 1996).

Kidney patients on dialysis must restrict their fluids to four cups per day. They can only have three ounces of square hard cheese per week and no soft cheese. Cream cheese is all right because it is lower in absorbable potassium. Margarine and mayonnaise is all right, and one teaspoon of jam is all right. For dialysis patients who are not diabetic, jam can be unlimited. The patient should eat three well-spaced meals a day and one snack. No chick peas, split peas, lentils, beans, or barley should be eaten. Bean sprouts are all right, but dried fruits are bad because they have too much potassium. White bread (*challah*) and light rye are the only types of bread that kidney patients can eat. Whole wheat is to be avoided. Bagels without seeds are all right and half a cup of coleslaw is all right, but no more than that. Nuts are bad, and so are seeds. Popcorn is all right without salt. Processed meats like bologna and salami are to be avoided, and corned beef is to be avoided. Steak, chicken, fish, and hamburger are all right. No ketchup, mustard, or relish should be eaten. Pizza without cheese is all right as long as it does not have too much tomato sauce and high-potassium fruits and vegetables as toppings. Also, the tomato sauce should be considered one of the high-potassium vegetables for the day. Chinese food is good, as well as green peas. Mixed vegetables are also low in potassium. No bran muffins, potato chips, baked potatoes, or popcorn with salt can be eaten. Plain muffins are all right.

Examples of high-potassium foods are apricots, avocado, banana, cantaloupe, honeydew melon, dried fruits, raisins, dates, figs, kiwi fruit, mangoes, nectarines, oranges, papaya, and prunes. Orange juice, carrot juice, mixed vegetable juice, tomato juice, and prune juice are high in potassium.

High-potassium vegetables are asparagus, dried beans, dried peas, lentils, beets, brussels sprouts, kale, kohlrabi, okra, parsnips, rutabagas, spinach, Swiss chard, sweet potato, yams, tomato, tomato sauce, winter squash, and rappini. Baked potato and french fries are so high in potassium that they should be avoided altogether. Chocolate, cocoa, licorice, molasses, maple syrup, maple sugar, malted milk, postum, ovaltine, nuts and seeds, salt substitute (potassium), potato chips, and brown sugar are also high in potassium.

Examples of low-potassium foods that a hemodialysis patient can eat four per day are apples and applesauce, blackberries, blueberries, cherries, fruit cocktail, grapefruit, grapes (fresh), canned mandarin oranges, peaches, pears, pineapples, plums, raspberries, rhubarb, strawberries, tangerines, and watermelon as well as apple juice, grapefruit juice, and pineapple juice.

Low-potassium vegetables are alfalfa sprouts, bean sprouts, green or wax beans, broccoli, cabbage, carrots, cauliflower, celery, kernel corn, half a corn on the cob, cucumber, lettuce, mushrooms, onion, green peas, green peppers, radish, summer squash, turnip, and zucchini. Also, dairy products are high in potassium, and no more than half a portion of these should be eaten per day (Patterson, 1996).

Psychological Aspects of Coping with Kidney Failure

Going into dialysis after a failed kidney transplant or after your own kidneys fail can be a very difficult disappointment (McGee, 1994, p. 2). For one thing, you have to be more careful with your diet, and you have to be prepared to spend four hours with a needle stuck in you three times per week.

It is a goal of therapy to help people cope with the problems associated with dialysis. Erythropoietin made a big contribution to the quality of life of kidney patients by increasing blood hemoglobin, the oxygen-carrying portion of the blood. Cyclosporine improved kidney patients' lives by decreasing the likelihood of rejection of a transplanted kidney (McGee, 1994, p. 2). Kidney patients and their caregivers form a team to try to improve the quality of life of kidney patients after kidney failure (McGee, 1994, p. 3).

The fact that end-stage renal disease (ESRD) is a formidable obstacle to overcome is evidenced by the high level of suicide among kidney patients (McGee, 1994, p. 3). Indeed, dialysis patients, by threatening not to go to dialysis, are similar to people pointing a loaded revolver to their heads. Because people attempt suicide younger when they are kidney patients, it is another indicator of the stress (psychological) of kidney failure. The failed transplant group felt the greatest hopelessness of all (McGee, 1994, p. 3). However, I have seen a patient who had three failed kidney transplants and is still coping with dialysis at age twenty-three. She first went into kidney failure when she was seven.

It has been my finding from working with suicidal patients and also from personal experience that suicidal tendencies are a combination of two factors. One is an intolerable situation, and the other is having no hope that the situation will get better. By removing the hopelessness, you can get rid of the suicidal tendency. That is one of the aims of this project: namely, to give hope. In order to give a definitive solution, you must make the offending situation more tolerable. When you give a person too many false hopes, eventually he stops believing in hope.

It is very difficult to cope with ESRD. My friend does very well to cope with her ESRD and stays in good spirits despite having some down moments and despite the fact that she does not always get good care from people close to her. I believe that this constitutes courage on her part. Among other kidney patients, I have seen anger and resentment as well as hopelessness. Different people have a different ability to react to chronic illness. I once had a nursing supervisor who said that mental health was the most important aspect of health. If you have your mental health, you have everything. This is another reason why we should keep up the quality of life of kidney patients. One suggestion by McGee and Bradley is to focus on aspects of life other than health, such as making money (1998, p. 4).

McGee and Bradley suggest cognitive-behavioural therapies as well as self-care to improve the quality of life of kidney patients (1998, p. 6). Cognitive-behavioural strategies mean strategies that involve changing the way we think and act. An example of cognitive therapy is to pinpoint things that we say to ourselves that make our mood negative, then write them down. Every human being talks to himself in one way or another, and the persons who are healthy and feel good are the persons who talk pleasantly to themselves. After writing down the bad thoughts, we must refute them and substitute logical good thoughts and self-statements for the bad thoughts so that we feel better. We must also look at behaviours that we want to change, write down our strengths and weaknesses, and write down steps that we want to take in order to make our personality what we want it to be. For example, someone may feel that he wants more strength and endurance, more education, and more assertiveness. He can write down a series of steps telling a hierarchy of ten to twelve behaviours that can be used to reach his goals. These behaviours should start from the easiest and move toward the more difficult.

In assessing the quality of life for kidney-failure patients, we must look at what the best treatment options are. We need good patient-professional interactions, especially with nurses and doctors, and we must prepare patients and health care staff for difficulties in the ESRD program. Most importantly, in order to improve the quality of life for kidney-failure patients, we can look at people who are coping well with kidney failure and find out what they are doing right (McGee, 1994, p. 10).

Studies have shown that spouses of ESRD patients often have as much difficulty coping as the actual ESRD patient. This indicates that they should involve themselves in the emotional therapy of patients (McGee, 1998, p. 36).

McGee found three factors affecting the survival of ESRD persons, with respect to spousal support. One of these is having a family that sticks together. Family accomplishment in terms of education, intellectual functioning, and household income were also important. Also, family integration and intactness was a factor (McGee, 1998, p. 36).

Psychological Conditions in ESRD

Kidney patients have a higher incidence of psychotic states, anxiety disorders, manic conditions, and most commonly, depression. One study reported that 60% of ESRD patients suffered from some form of depression (McGee, 1998 p. 37). This was evaluated by clinical psychiatric evaluation and objective tests, usually self-report inventories. In 1971, Akam, Moore, and Westevelt reported a suicide rate ten times that of the normal population (McGee, 1998, p.37). Stopping dialysis (considered suicide) accounted for twenty-two deaths among those studied (McGee, 1998, p. 38). Comorbidity such as diabetes tended to increase depression. Antidepressant medication was found to be very effective so that accurate diagnosis, as in any medical specialty, is important. Even though research on the psychosocial aspects of ESRD has improved over the years, the overwhelming conclusion by McGee and Bradley is that it is grossly understudied (McGee, 1998, p. 39).

Kidney failure sometimes has a component of a neurobehavioural syndrome. It sometimes includes mental sluggishness, drowsiness, impaired attention and concentration, impaired information processing, as well as diminished scores on IQ and memory tests. Although there is not enough testing done, many doctors say that there is mental impairment with ESRD (McGee, 1998, p. 104). My friend is still excellent at mathematics, and although she exhibits mood swings, she has shown little impairment in cognitive function. Dialysis markedly improves intellectual functioning in ESRD patients, and that is probably the reason why patients on dialysis do not exhibit too much impairment in cognitive function once they are dialysed. One man even went through medical school while he was taking dialysis therapy for kidney failure. Kidney transplantation has also been found to improve cognitive functioning in renal patients (McGee, 1998, p. 101). These findings might encourage patients to continue on with their dialysis regimens. High creatinine levels in the blood were found to diminish mental alertness (McGee, 1998 p. 101). Patients on continuous ambulatory peritoneal dialysis (CAPD) did even better than patients on haemodialysis in cognitive function tests. This might be an added advantage of CAPD over haemodialysis.

The greatest suffering for dialysis patients occurs when they must rely either on strenuous manual labour or cognitive functioning for their living. However, with proper control of kidney failure, this can be overcome.

For the sake of compliance, McGee advocates explaining the importance of medication in terms of the well-being of the patient. This is an important factor, as is attendance at dialysis (McGee, 1998, p. 116).

It is important for patients not to blame themselves for their illness, and it is also important not to blame others (McGee, 1998, p. 117). McGee and Bradley state that sometimes the best of attitudes in which no one is blamed will not help the patient adapt universally. Everyone is different in this regard. Patients must adapt a common-sense idea of their illness to help them cope. They must realize that they are not being punished and must have a coping strategy to help them cope with this threat to their health. Renal department staff should help the patient cope, and patient and staff must appraise this coping strategy from time to time (McGee, 1998, p. 118).

Shelton and Croyle have identified five factors around which perception of illness is located. These are identity, cause of an illness, consequences, time line, and cure (McGee, 1998, p. 118). Identity is the perception of the disease. Cause relates to how the patient perceives he contacted the disease. Consequences are the expected outcome of the disease. Time line is the perception of when the patient will get better, and cure is the perception of whether or not the patient thinks he will get better. My friend partially realises that the disease is caused by diabetes, which in turn was caused by obesity. She is not fully aware of all the consequences of the illness, but when someone in the dialysis unit dies, she worries that her life will be greatly shortened. She does not think that she will get better or that a cure will be found, but from what I have read of the work of Woods and Humes, there is good reason to be hopeful. That is why the bioartificial kidney will be discussed so thoroughly later in this work. My friend says that she will have to go to dialysis "forever and ever, until I am old and grey." It is best to have a realistic idea of ESRD and know that there is not yet a cure, but it is also not well-known that two doctors are close to what will amount to a cure. John Woods and David Humes estimate that the bioartificial kidney will be ready for implantation into humans in two and a half years and will be ready for widespread use five years after that (Humes, 1998,). Studies have shown that poor perceptions of the disease have lead to poor control (McGee, 1994, p. 120), especially when there is comorbidity such as diabetes. Diabetes is usually not well controlled when the patient does not perceive it accurately. This emphasises the importance of education and even self-education.

Patients taking blood pressure medication sometimes took it only when the blood pressure was perceived to be raised. This was based on a fallacy because you cannot feel what your blood pressure is. It is very dangerous for a kidney patient to miss any medication.

With regard to compliance to therapy, it was found that if patients are contacted weekly by telephone, they are more likely to comply with their regimen (McGee, 1998, p. 121). Faith in medical staff and the treatment they have to offer is also an important factor in compliance. It is also an important factor in coping with kidney disease—or any disease, for that matter.

Patient support groups are helpful in getting people to realize that there are other people with similar problems. It is also helpful to get people to realize the importance of compliance.

It was also found that adjustment of significant others was an important factor in adjusting to kidney disease (McGee, 1998, p. 123). People whose spouses or parents accepted their disease were more likely to have a better adjustment to their disease.

Vocational Rehabilitation

A study by Koch and Muthny using a large sample of kidney patients in Germany found that only a quarter of them were working steadily (McGee, 1998, p. 35). The sheer amount of time put in on dialysis is a deterrent by itself. Also, not feeling well a good part of the time would discourage working. I found that most of the patients in the dialysis unit were afraid to leave their disability pensions. McGee and Bradley found that the patients who did work were less depressed than their unemployed counterparts (McGee, 1998, p. 36). This was indicated by scores on the Beck Depression Inventory. One of the ways that my friend copes with the rigors of dialysis and the kidney regimen is by selling materials from her two businesses to nurses and patients. She also sells every time she gets some spare time. She hopes to get off her disability pension some day, although she was on her disability pension before she developed kidney trouble.

Studies have also shown that there is a decrease in social activities with ESRD. My friend on dialysis used to have a large circle of friends, but she has few friends now because she has alienated most of them with her mood swings and tiredness. I am really the only consistent friend that she has, and sometimes I am too busy to take her home and cook for her.

Sexual Adjustment

McGee and Bradley reported that few of the patients in studies regarding ESRD participated in sexual relations. There is a marked decrease in sexual desire and functioning in most kidney-failure patients due to fatigue and poor circulation as well as hormonal problems (McGee, 1998, p. 36). My friend and I have stopped having sexual relations since she got sick because she has not had the energy. McGee and Bradley report that support of loved ones causes patients to live longer (McGee, 1998, p. 36). My friend's decreased sex drive is not a problem because we can savour the experiences we do have and have had. Also, Ann Landers reports from a poll of readers that most people prefer cuddling to sex. Sex is not extremely important to many people.

Exercise

Exercise for ESRD patients has a positive effect on red blood cells, lowers blood pressure, normalises lipid and carbohydrate metabolism, as well as having other benefits on health such as increased oxygen uptake ability. A study was done by Kutner on exercise for ESRD patients. The only people excluded from the study were people with severe high blood pressure, congestive heart failure, heart disease, nerve pain, debilitating musculoskeletal diseases, and poor vision from diabetes. I find that walking with my friend is the best exercise, but she is limited by her lack of stamina (see Kutner, 1990, p. 79).

The exercise session conducted by Kutner lasted twenty-five minutes. Five minutes were for stretching and warm-up. Fifteen minutes were for light cardiovascular workout to 60% of maximum heart rate. Maximum heart rate is calculated by subtracting your age from 220.

Finally, there was a five minute warm-down. Recumbent bicycles were used, as were floor exercises and jogging on the spot. The patients did this two times per week with a hope that they would work out a third time on their own.

Some patients at Toronto Hospital dialysis unit who had dialysis in their arms were able to exercise for half an hour on a recumbent bicycle while still getting dialysed. They reported better self-image, increased wind, increased mental awareness, increased physical fitness, and an increased sense of well-being. They did not feel like they were sick (Kutner, 1990, p. 88).

Some patients eventually took part in a "Medical Mile"—running and walking supervised by doctors and nurses—and reported feeling good from it. Patients were encouraged to walk in the hallways and use a stationary bicycle in their rooms (Kutner, 1990, p. 89). This decreased their need for medication to lower blood pressure and helped them sleep. Insulin requirements were decreased, there was less need for blood transfusions to raise hemoglobin, and red blood cell count was increased (Kutner, 1990, p. 89).

Nissenson found that endurance training is an excellent way to begin rehabilitating dialysis patients. It consisted of continuous, repetitive light movements that work the heart and strengthen it. Examples are swimming, bicycle riding, running, stair-climbing, and shadow boxing (Nissenson, 1993, p. 333).

Studies have shown that endurance training has a number of benefits for normal individuals. The fat (lipid) profile improves, and cholesterol lowers. This lowers the risk for coronary heart disease. Exercise may also get blood moving, making it less likely to form an unwanted clot. It can not only lower blood pressure and weight but can also lower anxiety, tension, and depression (Nissenson, 1993, p. 333). Exercise can also reduce bone calcium wastage, increase cardiac output, and increase glucose tolerance (decrease the lack of ability to use insulin to metabolise glucose). These changes can improve life and life span in everyone, including ESRD patients.

There are drawbacks to exercise in ESRD patients. Patients with heart trouble can have their problem exacerbated (Nissenson, 1993 p. 334). Also, fluctuation in blood potassium is a serious problem with strenuous exercise. That is why walking is probably better than running for ESRD patients. Strenuous exercise can cause dangerous excesses of potassium, while after stopping, equally dangerous lowering of blood potassium can occur (Nissenson, 1993, p. 334).

Temporarily increased blood pressure during exercise can cause risk of stroke, which is aggravated by making the blood thicker with more red blood cells (Nissenson, 1993, p. 334). It appears that exercise programs for ESRD patients should be closely supervised.

Nissenson lists walking, swimming, cycling, and light weight lifting as the best forms of exercise for dialysis patients. He cautions against strenuous running and heavy weight lifting for the reasons mentioned above with regard to dangerous fluctuations in blood potassium. Nissenson, however, has even watched some dialysis patients finish marathons (1993, p. 335). This is exceptional and must be built up to slowly. It is also very encouraging.

Exercise can be used as a reward to patients who otherwise might not want to comply with a low-potassium diet and calcium-maintaining medications (Nissenson, 1993, p. 335). If the person does not like exercise, obviously this strategy will not work.

Optimising Long-Term Care of Renal Patients

McGee and Bradley state that the best way to improve the daily management of patients is to hand over as much of that management as possible to the patients themselves (McGee, 1994, p. 169).

Some functions only doctors can do, such as prescribing medications and prescribing dialysis. Some people cannot do dialysis themselves, but it is best to involve patients in decisions as much as possible.

The characteristics of a patient-centred consultation are:

(1) Identification of the patient's perception of what is happening as well as what is happening to his body (the disease process). This work helps that purpose. Relatives should be brought into this process as well. Listening to patients and relatives descriptions of their perceptions of the disease can help the doctor in diagnosis and treatment as well (McGee, 1994, p. 173).

(2) Both patients and families as well as health-care professionals should each give their perceptions of the disease. Differences of opinions should be ironed out, and this leads to improved care, improved quality of life for the patient, and improved compliance (McGee, 1998, p. 173).

(3) Patient and health professional should agree on what should happen and how (McGee, 1998, p. 174). Patients, families, and health professionals should negotiate the treatment rather than have the doctor do all the prescribing. Patients who do not get this patient-centred therapy should try to find a health care professional who would provide it.

Case Study

This is the story of a forty-eight-year-old white female. She first developed non-insulin dependent diabetes at age forty-four. At that point, there was a mild rising of her blood urea nitrogen and creatinine. It was called renal azotemia. She was referred to the diabetic clinic at Branson Hospital to try to help her with weight loss. The doctor determined that if she lost weight, the diabetes would be reversed. She had a weight problem ever since she was twenty-five years old. She started off at 130 pounds on a 5-foot 2-inch frame, and then built that up to 160 pounds. At that point, she developed high blood pressure and was put on a beta-adrenergic inhibitor for it. Beta-adrenergic inhibitors decrease the force with which the heart pumps by stopping some of the nerve stimulation from going through to the heart and other organs. Her blood pressure stayed reasonably normal at 140/90 and sometimes 130/80. The doctor who put her on the blood-pressure medication was dismayed to find that she gained thirty more pounds from eating too much and exercising too little. At that time she was in her thirties and maintained this state until her forties. She had only the high blood pressure as a medical problem, but in her early forties, her weight crept up to 200, then 210, then 216. It stabilised then lessened after that. When I would take her for three-mile walks, she would lose four pounds. For her, to walk three miles was similar to me carrying a canoe for three miles.

At age forty-two, her blood sugar started to rise, but she would not admit to being diabetic. She remained that way for a few months until her blood sugar got so high that she needed a medication to cause her pancreas to produce more insulin. She then admitted to being diabetic but refused to take measures to reverse it. Obesity causes diabetes by causing the body to need more insulin to service the fat cells. At the same time that she became diabetic, her kidney function started to go downhill for reasons most of the doctors were not sure. When she went to a kidney doctor, he found that the diabetes was the cause of the kidney problem and told her to lose 60 pounds from 210. She was so upset that she went on an eating binge. She asked her family doctor to send her to another kidney doctor, who determined from her blood work that her kidneys were functioning at 30 to 35 percent efficiency. She still did not realize that she was going into kidney failure until her kidney function went down to 20 percent. At that point, she had a vascular access operation on her left arm that joined an artery with a vein. This was in anticipation of her needing dialysis. She was forty-five years old. The doctor said that she would not need dialysis for a few months, and she started to lose weight to a small extent.

She also started to need several medications. She needed special vitamins for diabetics. She needed calcitriol, a hormone normally produced by the kidneys that raises blood calcium. She needed 1,000 mg calcium three times a day. She needed nifedipine, which is a calcium channel blocker that relaxes smooth muscle and so dilates blood vessels and lowers blood pressure. Calcium causes muscles to contract and so makes them tense. However, blood calcium is not specifically related to calcium at the molecular level that calcium channel blockers affect. She needed glyburide for her diabetes to lower her blood sugar. She also needed iron pills and erythropoietin to raise her level of hemoglobin and give her more energy.

Finally, this poor woman had to go on dialysis. There were no spots on dialysis open, so she had to go to the hospital, which she described as "prison camp." I visited her every day, and that was a great comfort for her and allowed her to get out for a walk. She went home to her parents every weekend and enjoyed getting out. She also enjoyed going for short walks a few times a day. She could not walk far because her hemoglobin was very low.

Everything went fairly well until the vascular access in her left arm became clotted, and she needed balloon angioplasty to unclot it. A needle was inserted into her arm near the graft. She was given Demerol to ease the pain. A plastic tube with a balloon in it was inserted to push the clot back into the vein. It worked for a few weeks and had to be repeated several times, causing great pain. Finally, the clots could not be gotten rid of and a catheter had to be inserted into her shoulder vein to perform dialysis from. Even this tended to get clots. Part of the reason for the clots was that diabetes tends to make blood clot. This is what ruined her kidneys. She had the same disorder in her kidneys that heart patients have in their hearts—namely, atherosclerosis. Inserting needles into a vein sets the clotting mechanism into motion. Also, she had small veins so that they tended to block easily.

She eventually had to have a vascular access operation in the other arm, higher up on the other arm, and then in a huge artery and vein in her leg. That operation held up for six months then needed declotting but is working all right now.

What got her through this was courage in terms of a will to live. She knew she had to have dialysis or die and did not give up. She felt that she could solve her problems with a kidney transplant but became apprehensive when she found out what that entailed. Here was a woman who disliked needles so much that she could barely stand to have blood taken, yet she submitted to dialysis without complaint. However, the thought of becoming an insulin-dependent diabetic was too much for her, as some of the antirejection drugs would do.

In terms of helping her cope emotionally with kidney failure and all it entailed, she enjoyed shopping and being taken to restaurants and plays and movies as much as possible. As long as her weekends were good, she could stand the weekdays. She still likes going for short walks but does not have the stamina to walk more than half a mile. She is cheerful most of the time but admits to feeling sorry for herself when she is alone, although I have not seen it. Her nurses feel that she is a Dr. Jekyll-Mr. Hyde personality who can be violent sometimes and sweet at other times. They praise her when she acts well. She has had a violence code called for her a few times because she has threatened other patients. Being a kidney patient is probably lonely and distressing for someone who does not have a caring partner. Also, when someone has a kidney transplant, they will need someone to look after them while they are recuperating from the operation. It is major and traumatic surgery. This woman in most ways is a model of how to cope with kidney failure.

Future of Kidney-Failure Research

The future of kidney-failure research is rapidly becoming the present. John Woods and David Humes are developing a bioartificial kidney that will one day do what a normal kidney does and will effectively be a cure for kidney failure. This research will take anywhere from two and one half years to two decades, but it looks very promising. There are a few other areas of research, but they are not as promising as the bioartificial kidney being created by these two researchers at the University of Michigan.

There are several reasons why a bioartificial kidney is needed. Among them are the fact that current treatments have too many problems associated with them. For example:

(a) Dialysis does not relieve symptoms completely.
(b) Dialysis is sometimes painful.
(c) Dialysis patients must restrict their fluid intake.
(d) Dialysis is time-consuming.
(e) If someone is unable to get to dialysis for too long, he will die.
(f) Restless people risk bleeding to death if they cannot sit still
(g) Dialysis patients have to watch potassium and phosphate intake.
(h) Dialysis patients have problems such as clotted vascular access, line catheter sepsis, and painful declotting procedures.

(i)   Dialysis patients have to take many medications in order to replace what their failed kidneys do not do.

(j)   Kidney transplants require antirejection drugs that damage the body.

(k)   A transplanted kidney only lasts eight to ten years.

(l)   Kidney transplant surgery is dangerous to some people.

(m)   Some people have their transplanted kidneys fail after two or three years, causing great psychological problems.

(n)   Being a transplant or dialysis patient causes psychological problems.

(o)   People on dialysis cannot vacation unless they are rich enough to afford dialysis away from home.

(p)   Kidney transplant patients are put through rigorous postoperative procedures such as having tubes running into and out of their bodies.

(q)   There is a lack of availability of suitable donor organs.

(r)   Dialysis does not replace making of calcitriol to control calcium balance. It gives limited excretion of potassium, it is an ordeal, it does not control blood pressure or metabolism, and it does not produce hormones. The patients on dialysis have major problems. (Schnermann, 1994, pp. 1-201).

What An Ideal Bioartificial Kidney Will Do

An ideal bioartificial kidney for one thing would filter out harmful substances in the blood so that the patient is detoxified of substances such as urea and creatinine. It would maintain water balance in the body. It would secrete necessary hormones such as erythropoietin, renin, and angiotensin 2 and excrete excesses of sugar, drugs, and other substances such as amino acids and organic positively and negatively charged particles. It would control thirst and allow unrestricted fluid intake. It would also maintain the acid-base balance of the body by excreting excess hydrogen ions and slowing down bicarbonate excretion, if necessary, or doing the opposite, if necessary. It would excrete excess sodium chloride (salt) and control sodium balance in the body as well as blood pressure. Above all, the patient could start urinating again, and the bioartificial kidney would hopefully last for the rest of the patient's long life span.

An ideal bioartificial kidney would bolster the patient's immune system by preventing destruction of white blood cells as well as allow the patient to have more energy. There would be less susceptibility to infection that is common among both kidney transplant patients and dialysis patients.

Are these goals feasible? I think that they will be accomplished sometime soon. David Humes has replaced the kidneys of small animals with bioartificial kidneys that do most or all of what a real kidney can do. Dr. Humes's assistant says that the bioartificial kidney must now be scaled up to implant into humans and will take approximately two and one half years. After five years of testing, if it is successful, mass production will be possible (taken from a recording in Dr. Humes's lab). The University of Michigan is the only place where research into a bioartificial kidney is being done. University of Toronto is looking into tissue engineering of a bioartificial heart.

How Will Bioartificial Kidneys Be Made?

Bioartificial kidneys will be made by a process called tissue engineering. This is done by using development of materials or devices capable of specific interaction with biological tissues. These combine novel materials with living cells to yield functional tissue equivalents (University of Toronto, p. 1). These tissues are useful for organ tissue replacement where there is a limited availability of donor organs, or where, in some cases, like nerves, no natural replacements are available. These constructs are also useful for the delivery of gene therapy. This would be very useful for diabetics because genetic disorders often cause diabetes which often causes kidney failure.

Tissue engineering can come in two guises: in one case cells are grown in culture and seeded onto a material, in another case an implanted material induces a specific response, such as tissue regeneration in living organisms (University of Toronto, p.1).

Tissue engineering exploits advances in a number of technologies, such as: biomaterials, drug delivery, recombinant DNA techniques in which the hereditary material, DNA is grown and alters the growth of living cells, biodegradable polymers, in which chemicals essential for life are broken down into their constituent parts, stem cell isolation, cell encapsulation (cell covering), and immobilisation of structures that hold up cells. It is also based on advances in the understanding of the features that control cell behaviour and wound healing, such as a matrix of materials outside cells, growth factors, and the immune system. Since tissue engineering involves the redoing of the steps involved in embryological development, this field can be considered a form of applied developmental biology (University of Toronto, p.1).

The bioartificial kidney will be made in a manner similar to the way an artificial pancreas or artificial liver would be made. Insulin producing cells or liver cells are microencapsulated in a polymeric membrane and transplanted as replacement organs. Because the cells are encapsulated, the host does not require antirejection drugs (University of Toronto, p.2). There are a number of other uses for tissue engineering, but we are mainly interested in the bioartificial kidney.

The kidney was the first organ to be transplanted and also was the first organ to have a machine made to replace its function, namely the dialysis machine (Humes, 1993, p. 678). It looks like the kidney will be the first solid organ to be successfully replaced with tissue engineering.

David Humes of the University of Michigan has already created an outside-the-body renal assistance device (RAD) for patients suffering from acute renal failure. It runs blood through a device outside the body but attached to the person in order to speed recovery. This device is hoped to be a step toward the ultimate goal, which is creating an implantable replacement organ for chronic renal failure. This device may at first extend the time between dialysis sessions for patients in chronic renal failure, and they hope to refine an implantable erythropoietin hormone-dosing device in order to overcome the low hemoglobin that kidney patients have. These endeavours are being undertaken by a private laboratory. Availability to patients of a bioartificial kidney is still some years away, but intermediate devices like the RAD are hoped to be deployed sooner (University of Michigan Health System, 1999, Humes, D. and Cutler, Dan).

Besides secreting hormones, the kidneys cleanse the blood in two steps. First, the blood is grossly filtered by driving the blood through a structure consisting of a tangled wall of capillaries, called the glomerulus. Under increased pressure, small molecules are driven out through the capillaries leaky walls. A great deal of water and other valuable small molecules are also filtered out in the process. All of this ultrafiltrate is captured and funnelled through a looping tube, whose walls are made of specialised cells. These cells have evolved to recapture the water and other "good" molecules and return them to general circulation, while leaving the waste to drain away to the bladder and be voided from the body (Humes, 1998, p. 1).

As we can see, filtration is a two step process, gross filtration, followed by selective reabsorption. Dialysis as it is now currently reproduces only step one, the gross filtration. The artificial kidney now used in dialysis is comprised of thousands of fine hollow fibers with permeable walls. The patient's blood laden with metabolic wastes, is diverted through the fibers. These are bathed in a fluid that draws off waste molecules.

This lifesaving treatment still leaves people with serious health problems (Humes, 1998, p.1).

The approach taken by David Humes's laboratory is to recreate the kidney's two-step filtration with an artificial two-step process. They are developing a filter to be linked in series with a reabsorbing unit. If both steps can be made efficient, the path will be clear to producing an implantable device (ibid, p.2).

A recent discovery in the laboratory of David Humes increased the feasibility of making a bioartificial kidney. Among the reabsorbing cells that comprised the wall of the looping tubule (Loop of Henle), are certain "stem" cells that retain a fetal-like capability of rapidly expanding and developing into specialised cells. David Humes's laboratory has created techniques for collecting these cells and expanding their numbers outside the body, making them available for incorporation into a reabsorbing device to replace the kidney tubule (Humes, 1998, p. 2).

The reabsorbing device begins with a porous hollow fiber, such as that used in the standard artificial kidney in a dialysis machine. The inner surface of this fiber is lined with living tubule cells, which are first precoated with a matrix to support cell growth. The cells arrange themselves in a natural array, forming a functioning tubule. Experiments have proven that the cells do function, reabsorbing ultrafiltrate at clinically useful rates (Humes, 1998, p. 2).

This discussion has so far addressed mostly the kidney's role in eliminating metabolic waste. Now is the time to discuss some other important functions of the kidney. The kidney, among other things is the body's chief regulator of red blood cells. Certain cells in the kidney sense the level of oxygen being delivered to the tissues. In response, these kidney cells produce and release into the bloodstream the hormone, erythropoietin (EPO). EPO stimulates bone marrow to produce red blood cells. When the kidney cells recognize adequate oxygenation in the tissues, they cease producing EPO (Humes, 1998, p.2). This is known as a feedback loop in which one situation affects another, and the other situation corrects the original situation. The goal is to create a steady state called homeostasis.

An individual in kidney failure loses the ability to monitor and adjust tissue oxygenation through red blood cell production. At this point, I would mention that red blood cells contain hemoglobin, a molecule containing iron, which transports oxygen throughout the body. Because the individual in kidney failure lacks EPO, they can become severely anemic, meaning lacking in red blood cells. If the anemia becomes too severe, which often happens when a kidney failure patient loses too much blood, they must get a blood transfusion. Regular injections of carefully calculated doses of EPO can ameliorate the anemia, but they are not as good as a natural kidney's feedback loop. Dr. Humes's laboratory is working on a method of incorporating the EPO-producing cells into the bioartificial kidney (Humes, 1998, p. 3).

Even without a perfect bioartificial kidney, an implantable filter alone would increase the length of time between dialysis sessions, possibly allowing the patient to need only one or two dialysis sessions a week. Other critical functions of the kidney, such as regulating blood pressure, producing renin and angiotensin 2, regulating calcium balance with calcitriol, maintaining sodium balance and maintaining integrity of the immune system, are hoped to be incorporated into the bioartificial kidney. This type of work falls within a rapidly evolving discipline called "tissue engineering"—the designing for manufacture of equivalents to living natural tissue. Tissue engineering is an exciting part of biomedical engineering (Humes, 1998, p. 3).

My original goal was to extrapolate from both a natural kidney and a dialysis machine in order to make an implantable artificial kidney. When I looked at kidney anatomy and physiology and how small and thin the functional unit of the kidney, the nephron was, and also studied the dialysis machine, I determined that an implantable artificial kidney was impossible. This idea was further strengthened by reading that an artificial kidney was impossible. I was furthered discouraged when this was confirmed by Edward Cole, MD, the transplant leader at Toronto Hospital. As a last try, I called Michael Sefton, head of biomedical engineering at University of Toronto, and he said that it is indeed feasible to make an artificial, implantable kidney through tissue engineering and that scientists at the University of Michigan were working on it. When I looked up the bioartificial kidney in the University of Toronto science library, I found about five or six articles written by Dr. John Woods and Dr. David Humes. I found that their work was more brilliant than I could have imagined and now I feel optimistic that a bioartificial kidney is indeed possible. There is a saying that "new problems cannot be solved by old ideas (Combden, 1998).

Obstacles to Developing a Bioartificial Kidney

1. It is unclear whether proximal tubule progenitor cells are able to differentiate into other kidney segment cells. The early indication is that they can (a) because they recover after acute injury and (b) because recovery can be made from acute tubular necrosis. Growth factors, TGF-B1 (tubular growth factor and EGF [extracellular

growth factor]), along with retinoid, the retinoic acid, promoted tubulogenesis in renal proximal tubule progenitor cells in tissue culture. This finding is one of the first definitions of inductive factors which may be important in making a mammalian organ (Humes and Cieslinski, 1993, pp. 678-678).

2. There needs to be considerable pressure to move the water and solutes from one part of a semipermeable membrane to another. The approach taken by Dr. Humes is to use heat and an electrical charge called convection to move particles from one end to another. Convective transport has been achieved outside living cells with the use of polysulphone hollow fibers.

3. Bleeding associated with required anticoagulation is a problem. In order to solve this problem, endothelial cell seeding of small-calibre vascular prostheses have been shown to reduce clotting. With regard to preventing clots, another avenue is open. Transferring genes into endothelial cells for the production of an anticoagulant protein that will work locally so that no bleeding is caused, is clearly conceivable (Humes, 1996, p. 2033).

4. These ideas can replace the need for anticoagulants, as well as preventing clots, which is the fourth obstacle to producing the bioartificial kidney (Humes, 1993, p. 678-679).

5. The fifth obstacle to producing a bioartificial kidney is rejection of foreign tissue. One of the solutions to this problem is to grow the biomaterials from the patient's own cells. Also, encapsulating foreign cells so that they do not contact cells of the body, such as circulating blood can eliminate the problem of rejection (Cutler, 1998).

6. A sixth obstacle to producing an effective bioartificial kidney is diminution of filtration rate due to protein deposition or clotting or both. This has been solved by using endothelial (inside the body) seeded conduits along filtration devices. Cells from the patient's body (usually blood vessel cells) are used to eliminate the problem of rejection of foreign tissue.

Illustrations

1. Normal kidney
2. Nephron
3. Hemodialyser
4. Kidney Transplant
5. Bioartificial Kidney

Normal Kidney

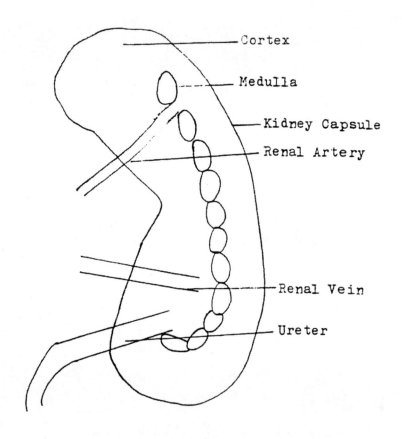

(Schnermann, 1998, p.13)

Nephron

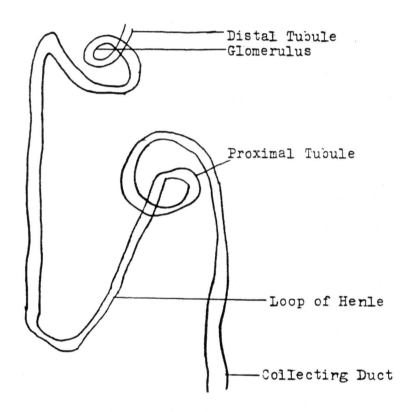

(Schnermann, 1998, p. 14)

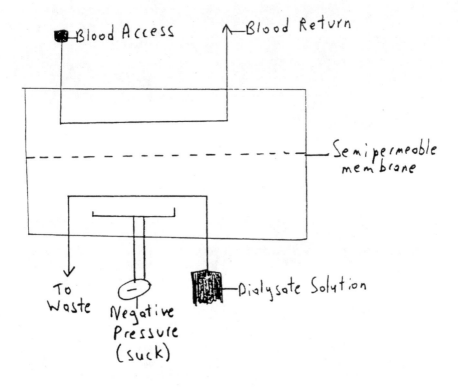

Blood Access

Blood Return

Semipermeable
membrane

To
Waste

Negative
Pressure
(suck)

Dialysate Solution

(Nissenson, 1992, p. 41)

Hemodialyser

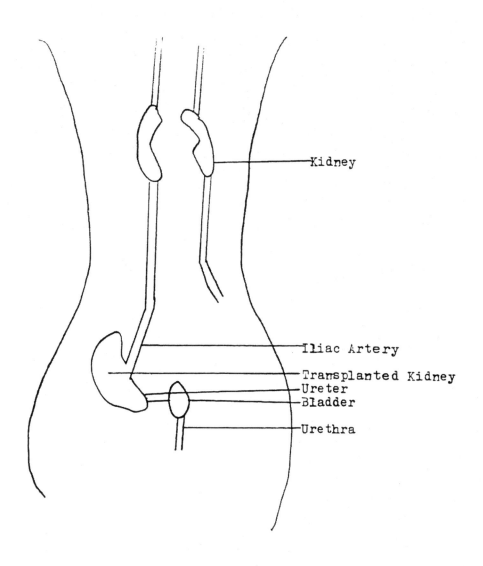

Kidney Transplant

(Toronto Hospital Kidney Transplant Manual, p.46)

Bioartificial Kidney

1.   Arterial blood delivered to kidney device.
2.   Endothelial cell-lined fibers filters blood.
3.   Filtrate delivered to re-absorbing device.
4.   Epithelial cells on inside of fibers re-absorb, and transport re-absorbate to extracapillary space.
5.   Re-absorbate added to circulation.
6.   Urine voided to bladder.
       (Humes, 1996, p. 385)

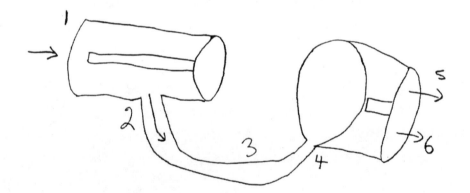

Bibliography

Abraham, Carolyn. Toronto Globe and Mail Newspaper. January 6, 1999, p. 1.

Cameron, Stewart. *Kidney Failure: The Facts*. N.Y.: Oxford University Press, 1996.

Cole, Edward, 1994, interview.

Cole, Edward 1996, interview.

Cole, Edward, 1998, interview.

Combden, Casey, December, 1998, interview.

Cotter, Lorna, February, 1998, interview.

Cutler, Daniel S. 1998 interview.

Douglis, Carole. *Inventions and Discoveries Changing Our World*. Washington, D.C. National Geographic Society, 1988.

Fisher, Craig and Wilcox, Christopher. *Nephrology*. Baltimore. Williams and Wilkins, 1993.

Fox, Cynthia. *Life Magazine*. Fall, 1998. p. 76.

Ganong, William. *Review of Medical Physiology.* Norwalk, Connecticut. Appleton and Lange 1995.

Gilmore, Ian, 1995, interview.

Humes, R. David and Cieslinski, R. Deborah. Tissue Engineering of a Bioartificial Kidney. *Biotechnology and Bioengineering.* Ann Arbour, Michigan. John Wiley and Sons, 1993.

Humes, R. David. Application of gene and cell therapies in the tissue engineering of a bioartificial kidney. *The International Journal of Artificial Organs.* Volume 19, No. 4, 1996. pp. 215-217.

Humes, R. David 1998a, interview.

Humes, R. David. 1998b, pamphlet.

Humes, R. David 1998c, recording in laboratory.

Humes, R. David and Cutler, Daniel S. *University of Michigan Health Systems, Inc.* Ann Arbour, Michigan, 1999.

Kutner, Mary. Sanders, Diane and Bower, John D. *Maximising Rehabilitation in Chronic Renal Disease.* N.Y. P.M.A. Publishing Corporation. 1990.

Lacome, Bernard, 1998, interview.

Locatelli, Francesco. Mortality and Morbidity on Maintenance Dialysis. *Nephron.* Volume 80, 1998. pp. 380-400.

Macdonald, Erica, dialysis nurse, 1998, interview.

McGee, Hannah and Bradley, Clare. *Quality of Life Following Renal Failure.* Berkshire, Great Britain. Harwood Academic Publishers. 1994.

McKnight, Teresa and McQuaine, Brenda. *Kidney Transplant Manual.* The Toronto Hospital. Multi Organ Transplant Program. TTH Publishing. 1997.

Macantoni, Carmelita. Progression of Renal Failure in Diabetic Nephropathy. *Nephrology, Dialysis, Transplant.* Volume 13, 1998. pp. 16-19.

McPhee, Stephen et al. *Pathophysiology of Disease.* Stamford, Connecticut. Appleton and Lange. 1997.

Mercer, Thomas H. Development of a walking test for the assessment of functional capacity in non-anaemic maintenance dialysis patients. *Nephrology, Dialysis, Transplant.* Volume 13, 1998. pp. 2023-2026.

Morell, Virginia. A Clone of One's Own, *Discover Magazine.* May, 1998.

Nissenson, Allen. *Dialysis Therapy.* Philadelphia. Hanley and Belfus, Inc. 1992.

Patterson, Jane, 1996, interview.

Pool, Robert. *Discover Magazine.* May, 1998, pp.52-7.

Reeves, Charlene. *Principles of Medical-Surgical Nursing.* N.Y. Lippincott, 1999.

Richardson, Sarah. *Discover Magazine.* January, 1999, pp.58-60.

Ritz, E. et al. The drama of the continuous increase in ESRF in patients with type 2 diabetes mellitus. *Nephrology, Dialysis, Transplantation.* Volume 13, 1998, pp.6-10.

Schena, F.P. New insights into therapy with monoclonal antibodies in allograft transplantation. *Nephrology, Dialysis, Transplantation.* Volume 12, 1997, pp. 55-8.

Schnermann, Jurgen. *Kidney Physiology.* N.Y. Lippincott, 1998.

Sedgewick, John. *Principles and Practices of Renal Nursing.* Cheltenham, U.K. Stanley Thomas Ltd. Publishers, 1998.

Toronto Star, Associated Press. Seoul, Korea, Dec. 17, 1998, p.1.

University of Toronto, Department of Biomedical Engineering Website. http://W.W.W.ibme.utoronto.ca/research/tissue. htm.

Wilmot, Ian. *Scientific American.* December, 1998, pp.58-63.

Edwards Brothers, Inc.
Thorofare, NJ USA
June 24, 2011